Seasonal
Patterns of
Hospital Activity

Seasonal Patterns of Hospital Activity

P. Joseph Phillip
Stephen J. Dombrosk
American Hospital Association

Lexington Books
D.C. Heath and Company
Lexington, Massachusetts
Toronto

Library of Congress Cataloging in Publication Data

Phillip, P. Joseph.
  Seasonal patterns of hospital activity.

  Includes index.
  1. Hospital utilization—United States—Seasonal variations—Statistics.
2. Hospitals—United States—Finance—Statistics. 3. United States—Statistics, Medical. I. Dombrosk, Stephen, joint author. II. Title. [DNLM:
1. Seasons—Statistics. 2. Hospitalization—Statistics. WX16 P557s]
RA981.A2P49   362.1'1'0973   79-1752
ISBN 0-669-02926-2

International Standard Book Number: 0-669-02926-2

Library of Congress Catalog Card Number: 79-1752

Contents

List of Figures

List of Tables

Preface

This book is based on the data collected, on a monthly basis, by the American Hospital Association and disseminated in the midmonth issue of the journal *Hospitals* under the caption "Hospital Indicators". These "hospital indicators," also known as "hospital statistics," appear in the journal in their raw form; that is, they are not adjusted for seasonal fluctuations in the level and tempo of activity experienced by hospitals. However, raw data are useful and important in their own right, and the journal will continue the publication of the indicators in that form.

The seasonal indexes presented in this book offer an easy way of "deseasonalizing" the indicators, that is, correcting the indicators for seasonal fluctuations. All that must be done is to divide the raw monthly value of an indicator by the appropriate seasonal index. There is a variety of situations where deseasonalized values provide a better perspective on the true situation than raw values. Indeed, raw values can at times be confusing and even misleading if used out of context. For example, the seesaw pattern that characterizes the monthly movement of raw data makes it difficult to discern underlying trends. For the same reason, generalizations made on the basis of the latest available raw data are apt to be misleading. For instance, if the latest available raw data pertain to the month of December, expenses per day would seem deceptively high, and occupancy rate would seem deceptively low. Similarly, births and related newborn utilization measures are abnormally high during the fall and abnormally low during the spring, outpatient visits are abnormally high during the summer and abnormally low during the winter, and so on.

The first chapter introduces the hospital indicators published monthly in *Hospitals,* the Journal of the American Hospital Association. Some distinctive features of hospital indicators are also highlighted in this chapter.

Chapter 2 is devoted to an explanation of key hospital indicators, especially those developed in recent times as a sequel to the changing complexion of hospital care. Not only are these indicators defined, but their precise significance—what they really are as opposed to what they are sometimes taken to be—is spelled out in a manner that would, hopefully, lead to a better understanding and appreciation of the unique attributes of the hospital industry. We commend this chapter to those who are not intimately familiar with the statistics of the hospital industry.

The concept of seasonal variations, the factors that cause these variations, the effect of these variations on the monthly values of an indicator, and the definition of seasonal indexes constitute the subject matter of chapter 3.

The next chapter is devoted to a detailed demonstration of the various possible uses of seasonal indexes. These include the deseasonalization process, trend analysis, forecasting, estimation of annual totals from monthly values, assessment of facilities and resource needs, and so on. Wherever appropriate, simple worked-out examples are provided for the benefit of those unfamiliar with time-series analysis. The last section of this chapter summarizes the more important interrelationships among hospital indicators.

The seasonal patterns of twenty-three measures that include all the important statistics traditionally generated in the hospital industry are examined in this book. The index values and graphs pertaining to each of these measures are presented in chapter 5. The factors that contribute to the seasonal variations of each indicator and the manner in which the seasonal variations of an indicator impinge upon others are also examined in detail in this chapter.

The causes and consequences of regional differences are explored in chapter 6. It has been found, for example, that certain hospital utilization measures such as births, outpatient visits, and surgical operations are more sensitive than others to differences in climatic, topographic, demographic, socioeconomic, and institutional characteristics.

Presented in chapter 7 are the seasonal indexes for the nation as a whole and each of the nine census regions. Since there are ten regions and twenty-three hospital indicators, the number of index values presented total 10 X 23 X 12 = 2,760. This chapter also suggests ways in which users can determine whether the regional indexes provided in this book are applicable to their specific area of interest.

The nature of time series and the methodology employed for the construction of seasonal indexes are discussed in the appendixes. The formulas of all hospital statistics included or referred to in the text appear in the glossary.

It is hoped that the seasonal indexes presented in this book; the generalizations made therefrom concerning the pattern of hospital utilization, the behavior of revenue, expenses, capacity utilization, and so on; and the analysis of inter-regional differences would prove useful to hospital management; metropolitan and state hospital associations; health systems agencies; insurance carriers; local, state, and federal government agencies; and planners, researchers, and students in the health care field.

This book is written primarily for the lay audience. Therefore, concepts, procedures, and examples are elaborated to a degree which may seem, at times, superfluous to professional statisticians and researchers. However, inasmuch as potential users of the material in this book come from a variety of disciplines and backgrounds, we do hope that this approach will pay off in terms of a much broader readership.

The authors wish to express their appreciation to the reviewers of an earlier draft, Paul J. Feldstein, Ph.D., University of Michigan, Charles D. Flagle, Dr. Eng., Johns Hopkins University Hospital, and John Gaffney, Ph.D., American

Medical Association for their suggestions and constructive criticisms. They are, of course, not responsible for any errors of omission or commission.

Finally, we wish to thank the American Hospital Association and, in particular, Howard Berman, Vice President, for his advice, encouragement and, above all, forbearance in permitting us to devote as much time as we did to this project.

Seasonal Patterns of Hospital Activity

1

Introduction

In 1963 the American Hospital Association instituted the National Hospital Panel Survey[1] to gather monthly data on facilities, utilization, revenue, expenses, personnel, and so on pertaining to community hospitals.[2] The "hospital indicators" that appear monthly in *Hospitals,* journal of the American Hospital Association, are based on the data gathered through the Panel Survey. These indicators provide the latest information on various aspects of the performance of the industry, and they are recognized and used as such by member institutions; allied health associations; intermediaries; local, state, and federal agencies; the media; and the general public.

Like most periodic statistics we are familiar with, hospital indicators are subject to seasonal (monthly) fluctuations. The level and tempo of activity in hospitals are high during certain months of the year; they are low in certain other months. These variations are reflected in utilization indicators such as adjusted patient days,[3] adjusted admissions,[3] adult daily census[4] and occupancy rate. They are generally high during the early part of the year and low during the later part. The solid line of figure 1-1 depicts the monthly movements of adjusted patient days in 1975.[5] Notice the seesaw pattern. Aggregate financial indicators such as total revenue and total expenses move in concert with adjusted patient days. This is understandable because revenue and expenses are positively related to the volume of services provided. The higher the volume (that is, the higher the adjusted patient days), the higher will be the total revenue and total expenses.

The standardized measure, adjusted expenses per inpatient day (the broken line in figure 1-1), on the other hand, traces a pattern which is, more or less, the reverse of the pattern displayed by the volumetric utilization measure, adjusted patient days. Why is this so? A typical hospital has a high proportion of "fixed costs," that is, costs incurred for the maintenance and/or operations of buildings, fixtures, facilities, machinery, equipment, and so on. These costs remain, more or less, unchanged regardless of the volume of services provided. Consequently, when the volume of services—adjusted patient days—rises, adjusted expenses per inpatient day decline, and vice versa.

The reverse pattern just noted, which also applies to other standardized expense measures and volumetric measures of utilization, such as adjusted expenses per inpatient day versus adult daily census, adjusted expenses per admission versus admissions, and so on, is a ubiquitous feature of the hospital industry. The reason is that hospitals must, willy-nilly, maintain a certain "level of pro-

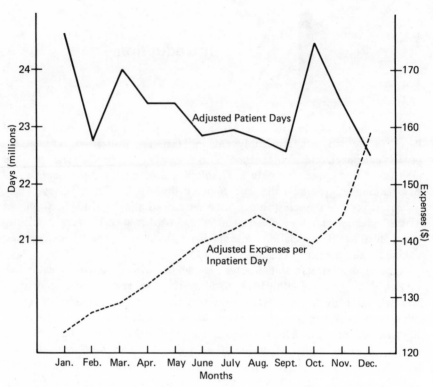

Figure 1-1. Adjusted Patient Days and Adjusted Expenses per Inpatient Day, 1975

tection," that is, empty beds, in order to deal with fluctuations in the demand for their services. What ought to be the optimum protection level continues to be a matter of controversy because it involves the reconciliation of two opposing goals—economic efficiency and the effectiveness of hospitals as providers of health care. It is easy to show that whenever a hospital reduces its protection level in an attempt to cut costs, its ability to meet community demand promptly and effectively is reduced *pro tanto*.[6]

There is an interesting relationship between length of stay and per diem expenses: the shorter the stay, the higher the expense per day.[7] This relationship is best explained in terms of the types of services a patient receives in an inpatient setting. These include (1) admission-specific services, such as x-ray examinations, blood tests, and so on, administered on the day the patient enters the hospital or immediately thereafter; (2) diagnoses-specific services, such as laboratory tests, diagnostic radiology procedures, and operating room services, which taper off toward the recovery phase of a patient's stay; and (3) stay-specific services, such as room and board and floor nursing, which remain, more or less, uniform over the days the patient stays in the hospital. It is now easy to see that "service intensity," that is, the quantity of routine and ancillary services provided per day, will be high if the length of stay is short. For example, expenses per day are likely to be rather high for diagnoses such as uterine fibroma (ICDA8:218) and disorders of menstruation (ICDA8:626), with average lengths of stay of less than 3 days. In contrast, expenses per day are likely to be low for a diagnosis such as malignant neoplasm of trachea, bronchus and lung (ICDA8:162), which has an average length of stay of over 20 days.

Unlike inpatient utilization, which tends to be high during winter, outpatient utilization is high during spring and summer. This is particularly so in the more urbanized areas of the country, such as census regions 1 (New England), 2 (Middle Atlantic), and 4 (East North Central). A possible explanation is the higher incidence of injuries resulting from accidents and crimes during the spring and summer months when people spend more time outdoors engaging in sports, recreation, and travel.

Certain indicators display patterns of their own. An instance in point is births and two related indicators, newborn days and newborn occupancy rate (see figure 1-2). These indicators are characterized by a trough in the spring and a peak in the fall. Studies focusing on the causes that underlie seasonal variations in births have generally placed "climatic conditions" at the head of the list. Takahashi, for example, found that conception rates varied roughly with temperature, with peaks in the conception rate from winter through spring to summer as one moves from countries of the Torrid Zone to the Northern Subfrigid Zone. He suggested that the pronounced downswing in the conception curve is greater in the South region during July and August because of the hot and humid climate during this period.[8] Striking evidence of this is provided in chapter 6 through a juxtaposition of the seasonal patterns of births for the nation and the East South Central region.

Finally, a note on the indicators pertaining to the month of February. Relatively speaking, February is a month in which the volume and tempo of activity are high. This is reflected in the high February values of indicators reflecting capacity utilization, such as adult daily census and occupancy rate. However, since February has only 28 days (except leap year), indicators pertaining to volumetric measures are low for this month. The "February dip" which seems to break the general pattern of these indicators is, in reality, caused by the shortness of the month. Since the indexes are constructed from the data pertaining to a 14-year period (including leap years), the February indexes have a slight bias. More specifically, the February indexes of the thirteen volumetric measures such as inpatient days, admissions, outpatient visits, total expenses, and so on are slightly overstated for standard years and understated for leap years. In contrast, the February indexes of adjusted expenses per inpatient day and revenue per adjusted patient day are slightly understated for standard years and overstated for leap years. (see table 5-1).

This book presents the seasonal indexes of a variety of hospital indicators,

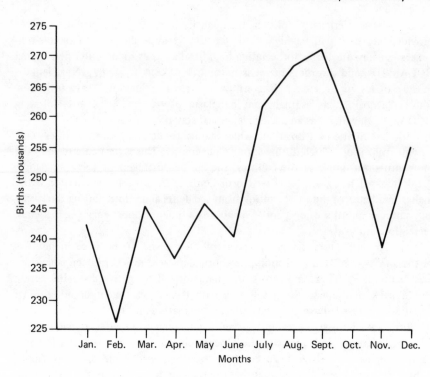

Figure 1-2. Births, 1975

some of them well known and some others not so well known. The next chapter is devoted to a discussion of those hospital indicators whose precise significance may not be readily apparent to some readers.

Notes

1. The panel consists of approximately 1,200 hospitals. The design is stratified random sampling with optimum allocation. Since beds are highly correlated with most of the indicators, the intrastratum variances of beds are used as the basis of allocation.

2. Community hospitals are defined as all nonfederal, short-term general and "other special" hospitals. "Other special" hospitals include the following services: obstetrics and gynecology; eye, ear, nose, and throat; rehabilitation; orthopedic; chronic disease; children's; and all other specialty services. Community hospitals represent 84 percent of all hospitals and account for 93 percent of all admissions in the United States.

3. There are six indicators in this book where the word *adjusted* appears as part of the name: adjusted admissions, adjusted patient days, revenue per

adjusted admission, revenue per adjusted patient day, adjusted expenses per admission, and adjusted expenses per inpatient day. These indicators should not be mistaken for *seasonally adjusted values.* The word *adjusted* as used in these instances refers to the fact that these indicators include outpatient visits. See chapter 2.

4. In the cases of the three indicators which contain the word *adult* in their names, it should be borne in mind that these include pediatric statistics. The only age group excluded is the newborn.

5. The raw values used in figure 1-1 and elsewhere in this book are taken from the "Hospital Indicators" that appear monthly in *Hospitals,* journal of the American Hospital Association. Reprinted with permission.

6. See, for example, P.J. Phillip. "Some Considerations Involved in Determining the Optimum Size of Specialized Hospital Facilities," *Inquiry* IV (December 1969): 44–48.

7. See, for example, U.S. Department of Health, Education and Welfare, S.S.A. *Selected Charge Pattern in Short-Stay Hospitals under Medicare,* No. HI-31, Sept. 30, 1971, Chart B.

8. E. Takahashi. "Seasonal Variation of Conception and Suicide," *Tohoku Journal of Experimental Medicine* 84 (Dec. 1964).

2

Significance of Selected Indicators

Most of the hospital indicators reported in this book have been around for many years and their meaning and significance are well understood by those associated with the hospital industry. However, the changing complexion of hospital care has necessitated the development of new statistics, such as adjusted patient days, adjusted expenses per inpatient day, adjusted expenses per admission, and so on. These statistics are not so well known, and their significance is sometimes misunderstood. Therefore, this chapter is devoted to a review of these statistics, with particular emphasis on their true significance and the reasons for their development.

Utilization Indicators

Some idea of the breadth and complexity of services offered by the modern hospital can be gained from the number of distinct facilities/services. The American Hospital Association's *Guide to the Health Care Field* (1977 ed.) lists fifty-one such facilities/services. Thus, in a real sense, hospitals are multiproduct firms providing a wide variety of services for the specialized needs of patients. However, in order to simplify the measurement of hospital output, hospitals are generally characterized as dual-product firms providing services in inpatient and outpatient settings.

The Concept of "Adjusted" Patient Days/Admissions

In the 1940s and 1950s, the American Hospital Association (AHA) reported two sets of statistics as measures of hospital utilization: inpatient days, or simply patient days, and admissions.[1] These two statistics are alternative ways of measuring the volume of hospital utilization inasmuch as admissions equal patient days times length of stay.

By the early 1960s it became all too obvious that patient days and admissions were not enough to express the volume of services because they ignored outpatient (ambulatory) services altogether. In 1962 the AHA introduced a third utilization statistic—outpatient visits—where the term *visits* refers to the appearance of outpatients in any unit of the outpatient department.

Figure 2-1 portrays the burgeoning growth of outpatient services over the

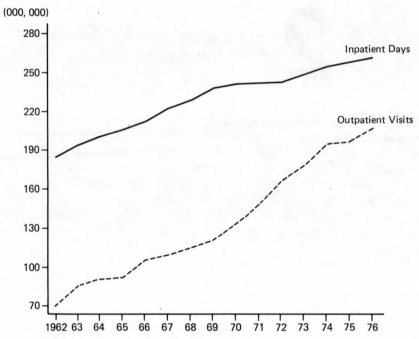

Source: American Hospital Association, *Hospital Statistics,* 1971 and 1977 eds. Reprinted with permission.

Figure 2-1. Growth Patterns: Inpatient Days and Outpatient Visits

past 14 years. In 1976, community hospitals handled 207.7 million outpatient visits compared with 70.7 million in 1962.[2] This represents a compounded annual growth rate of 8 percent, compared with a rate of 2.4 percent for inpatient days during the same period.

The recognition of outpatient services as a major product of the hospital industry gave rise to a new problem: How does one measure the total output of hospitals? An outpatient visit entails less resource use and is, therefore, less expensive than an inpatient day. Consequently, it becomes difficult to measure changes in the total output produced over time or across hospitals if the inpatient-outpatient mix varies. Consider, for example, the output of two hypothetical hospitals shown below:

Hospital	Annual Inpatient Days	Annual Outpatient Visits
Hospital A	40,000	5,000
Hospital B	36,000	30,000

Which of these hospitals has the larger output? It is difficult to say. The same difficulty arises when one attempts to compare changes in the output of a hospital or the industry between two time periods, say 1970 and 1975.

These problems can be resolved if a way is found to express the output of hospitals in some standardized units. For example, if the resource use involved in one inpatient day equals the resource use involved in, say, five outpatient visits, we could count five outpatient visits as equivalent to one inpatient day. This is the rationale behind adjusted patient days which have appeared in the later issues of *Hospital Statistics*.[3] Returning to our example, the adjusted patient days of hospitals A and B would be as follows:

$$\text{Hospital } A: \quad 40,000 + \left(\frac{5,000}{5}\right) = 41,000 \text{ adjusted patient days}$$

$$\text{Hospital } B: \quad 36,000 + \left(\frac{30,000}{5}\right) = 42,000 \text{ adjusted patient days}$$

Thus we are able to determine that hospital B has the larger volume of output.

A similar procedure is used to convert outpatient visits to *equivalent* admissions. For example, if the admissions of hospitals A and B are 5,000 and 4,500, respectively, and if the resource use involved per admission equals the resource use involved in, say, forty outpatient visits, adjusted admissions would be:

$$\text{Hospital } A: \quad 5,000 + \left(\frac{5,000}{40}\right) = 5,125 \text{ adjusted admissions}$$

$$\text{Hospital } B: \quad 4,500 + \left(\frac{30,000}{40}\right) = 5,250 \text{ adjusted admissions}$$

For the actual computation of adjusted patient days/admissions, the revenue derived from inpatient and outpatient services are used as proxies of resource use. Thus

$$\text{Adjusted patient days} = \text{inpatient days}$$
$$+ \text{ outpatient visits}\left(\frac{\text{revenue per outpatient visit}}{\text{revenue per inpatient day}}\right)$$

$$\text{Adjusted admissions} = \text{admissions}$$
$$+ \text{ outpatient visits}\left(\frac{\text{revenue per outpatient visit}}{\text{revenue per admission}}\right)$$

Expense Indicators

The accountants define *expenses* as expired costs. However, in the hospital industry, expenses and costs are generally used as synonyms. The American
Hospital Association publishes three expense statistics: total expenses, adjusted
expenses per inpatient day, and adjusted expenses per admission.

The Concept of "Adjusted" Expenses
per Inpatient Day/Admission

Adjusted expenses per inpatient day/admission are defined as follows:

$$\text{Adjusted expenses per inpatient day} = \frac{\text{total expenses}}{\text{adjusted patient days}}$$

$$= \frac{\text{total expenses}}{\text{inpatient days} + \text{outpatient visits}\left(\dfrac{\text{revenue per outpatient visit}}{\text{revenue per inpatient day}}\right)}$$

$$\text{Adjusted expenses per admission} = \frac{\text{total expenses}}{\text{Adjusted admissions}}$$

$$= \frac{\text{total expenses}}{\text{admissions} + \text{outpatient visits}\left(\dfrac{\text{revenue per outpatient visit}}{\text{revenue per admission}}\right)}$$

These expense statistics can be readily seen as corollaries of the adjusted utilization measures described earlier. However, as we shall see presently, they have
more significance than that.

Cost allocation by product line is a difficult undertaking for multiproduct
firms. This is particularly so for hospitals because of the commingling of resources that go into the production of inpatient and outpatient services. Consequently, hospitals seldom maintain separate cost centers for inpatient and
outpatient services, nor do they attempt to estimate and report separately the
expenses attributable to these products. What they report is a single expense
measure—total expenses.

Until 1962 the American Hospital Association reported two expense statistics, expenses per patient day and expenses per admission. These measures
were obtained by dividing the total expenses incurred by hospitals during a
year by the total patient days and admissions respectively during that year. For
example, in 1950 community hospitals incurred a total expense of $2.12 billion

and provided 135 million patient days, so expense per patient day worked out to $2.12 billion ÷ 135 million = $15.70 per patient day.

With the rapid growth of outpatient services, a substantial portion of the total expenses of hospitals pertains to the expenses incurred for outpatient care. It is therefore clearly incorrect to divide total expenses by patient days and call the resulting value expenses per patient day. For example, if 15 percent of total expenses pertains to outpatient care, then expenses per patient day computed in this way is overstated by 15 percent. Furthermore, since outpatient visits are rising at a faster pace than inpatient days, the rate at which expenses per patient day is rising would seem faster than it really is.

It is against the preceding background that the expense statistics introduced in 1963 by the American Hospital Association, adjusted expenses per inpatient day and adjusted expenses per admission, should be evaluated. They constitute an attempt to estimate the expenses attributable to inpatient care in a situation where inpatient-specific expense data are unavailable.

Adjusted expenses per inpatient day and adjusted expenses per admission are sometimes misunderstood as the averages of two products—a high-priced inpatient service and a low-priced outpatient service. This is certainly not so. Adjusted expenses per inpatient day is an *estimate of expense per patient day*. Likewise, adjusted expenses per admission is an *estimate of expenses per admission*. Perhaps this point can be driven home by demonstrating the equivalence between the formulas given earlier for adjusted expenses per inpatient day/ admission and the alternative formulas that follow:[4]

$$\text{Adjusted expenses per inpatient day} = \frac{\text{total expenses}\left(\dfrac{\text{inpatient revenue}}{\text{total patient revenue}}\right)}{\text{inpatient days}}$$

$$\text{Adjusted expenses per admission} = \frac{\text{total expenses}\left(\dfrac{\text{inpatient revenue}}{\text{total patient revenue}}\right)}{\text{admissions}}$$

It is clear from the preceding formulas that adjusted expenses per inpatient day/ admissions can be obtained by removing from total expenses an estimate of expenses incurred for outpatient services and dividing the remainder by inpatient days/admission.

Finally, if it is necessary to compute adjusted expenses per outpatient visit, the appropriate formula would be:

$$\text{Adjusted expenses per outpatient visit} = \frac{\text{total expenses}\left(\dfrac{\text{outpatient revenue}}{\text{total patient revenue}}\right)}{\text{outpatient visits}}$$

Revenue Indicators

Hospital revenue has two components: patient revenue and nonpatient revenue. The sum of these constitutes total revenue. Hospital revenue may also be broken down into (1) gross revenue, and (2) net revenue (that is, gross revenue less deductions for contractual adjustments, bad debts, charity, and so forth). The National Hospital Panel Survey gathers data on net revenue. As such, the revenue measures that constitute the basis of several indexes presented in this book are net revenue measures.

Revenue per Adjusted Patient Day/Admission

These statistics are computed as follows:

$$\text{Revenue per adjusted patient day} = \frac{\text{total revenue}}{\text{adjusted patient days}}$$

$$\text{Revenue per adjusted admission} = \frac{\text{total revenue}}{\text{adjusted admissions}}$$

Alternative Formulas

There are several alternative ways of computing these and other statistics reported in this book. See the glossary for a list of these formulas.

Year-End Beds and Statistical Beds

The American Hospital Association gathers data on beds in two ways: year-end beds and statistical beds. As the name implies, year-end beds is a count of the number of beds set up and staffed for use at the end of the year. Most hospitals have some latitude (albeit a limited one) to add or withdraw beds in response to short-run fluctuations in demand for inhospital care. The statistical beds reported annually in *Hospital Statistics* are weighted averages of the number of active beds that were available during the year. For example, assume that a hospital had 100 beds at the beginning of the year. In July it added 10 beds, but in October it withdrew 40 beds. Then the statistical beds for the year would be:[5]

$$100 + 6/12(10) - 3/12(40) = 95 \text{ beds}$$

The seasonal indexes of beds presented in this book pertain to statistical beds.

Notes

1. Discharges," "cases," and "episodes" are generally used as interchangeable expressions of "admissions" in short-stay hospitals. In long-term institutions, this practice will lead to substantial bias. See S. Falk, "Average Length of Stay in Long-Term Institutions," *Health Services Research,* 6 (Fall 1971): 251–255.

2. American Hospital Association, *Hospital Statistics,* 1972 ed. and 1977 ed. Reprinted with permission.

3. See, for example, American Hospital Association, *Hospital Statistics,* 1977 ed., Table 5A.

4. Proof (using symbols given in the glossary) is as follows: Since $TPR = IPR + OPR$, we may rewrite the formula for AED given in the text as follows:

$$AED = \frac{TE}{IPD} \cdot \frac{IPR}{TPR} = \frac{TE}{IPD} \cdot \frac{IPR}{(IPR + OPR)} = \frac{TE}{IPD} \cdot \frac{IPR}{IPR\left(1 + \dfrac{OPR}{IPR}\right)}$$

Cancelling out IPR from the numerator and the denominator of the expression on the extreme right, we have

$$AED = \frac{TE}{IPD\left(1 + \dfrac{OPR}{IPR}\right)} = \frac{TE}{IPD + \left(\dfrac{IPD \cdot OPR}{IPR}\right)} = \frac{TE}{IPD + \left(\dfrac{IPD}{IPR}\right)OPR}$$

Since $IPR = IPD \cdot RPD$, $IPD/IPR = 1/RPD$. And, $OPR = OPV \cdot ROPV$. Therefore,

$$AED = \frac{TE}{\left[IPD + \left(\dfrac{1}{RPD}\right)(OPV \cdot ROPV) \right]}$$

Rearranging terms, we have

$$AED = \frac{TE}{IPD + OPV\left(\dfrac{ROPV}{RPD}\right)} \qquad \text{Q.E.D.}$$

5. An alternative formula is:

$$\text{Statistical beds} = \sum_{1}^{n} W_t B_t$$

where B_t = number of beds available during period t

W_t = period t expressed as a fraction of total period (usually 12 months)

Thus for the present example

Statistical beds = $100(6/12) + 110(3/12) + 70(3/12)$

= 95 beds

3 Seasonal Variations

Like most indicators we are familiar with, such as the gross national product (GNP), the Dow-Jones industrial averages, unemployment rate, and so on, the movements of hospital indicators over time are influenced by several factors. These are discussed in some detail in appendix I. This chapter is devoted to a discussion of one of these factors, seasonal variations.

By *season variations* we mean variations that repeat themselves with a degree of regularity. Depending on the nature of the indicator, these variations could be hourly, daily, weekly, monthly, or quarterly. However, since monthly variations are more common and easier to deal with, seasonal variations are usually studied on a monthly basis. The term *seasonal variations* as used in this study means *monthly variations.*

Causes of Seasonal Variations

What are the causes that underlie seasonal variations? Climatic conditions such as rainfall, cold, snow, heat, sunshine, humidity, and smog cause variations in demand. So do social, cultural, and institutional factors such as holidays, vacation seasons, and production cycles. For example, hospital administrators are aware that inpatient activities are generally high during the winter months when people are exposed to inclement weather. Outpatient activities, particularly those resulting from accidents and violence, on the other hand, tend to be high during summer months when people spend more time outdoors. Finally, hospital activities slack off during December, a month in which people (including hospital personnel) combine vacations with holidays to participate in yule-related festivities.

When seasonal variations are present, the movement of an indicator exhibits a seesaw pattern as shown in figure 3-1. According to this graph (which is drawn for illustrative purposes only), the level of activity is at its peak during the month of January. June, September, and November are also months in which the levels of activity are high. In contrast, the level of activity reaches its lowest point during the month of December. February, March, July, and October are also months in which the levels of activity are low.

Seasonal patterns are of two kinds—stationary and nonstationary. A stationary pattern implies that the monthly ups and downs noticed in the past will remain stable over the years. For example, if January 1960 had been a month of

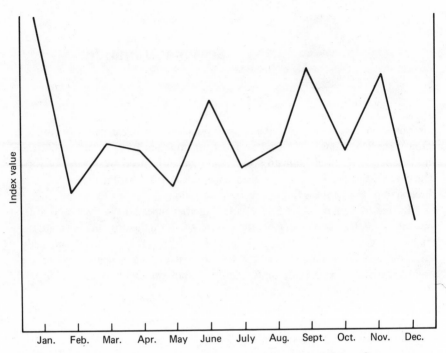

Figure 3-1. Seasonal Pattern: A Hypothetical Example

relatively brisk activity, this feature persists in January 1961, January 1962, and so on. In the case of a nonstationary pattern, the monthly ups and downs noticed in the past shift over time. This shift may be gradual, abrupt, or erratic. Most indicators in the economy are of the stationary kind, although there may be differences in the amplitude of monthly fluctuations observed over time. The kind of seasonal pattern and the degree to which the amplitude of monthly fluctuations remains constant may be ascertained by analyzing historical data pertaining to several years. Our analysis of data for the 14-year period (1963–1976) reveals that hospital indicators have stationary seasonal patterns, and that monthly fluctuations do exhibit a satisfactory degree of constancy (see appendix II).

Although this book focuses on monthly fluctuations, it should be emphasized that seasonal fluctuations can be studied in terms of periods other than a month. Much depends on the nature of the indicator and the purpose at hand. For example, it may be that, for certain indicators, seasonal fluctuations are more pronounced or more revealing if a time period other than a month is used. Also, the purpose sought to be achieved oftentimes dictates the appropriate time period. For instance, a hospital that plans to deploy personnel in its emergency department may want to study hourly fluctuations in the arrival of emergency cases.

Consider, for example, the seasonality of surgical operations presented in figure 5-19 (p. 64). Although this indicator does exhibit monthly variations, the general configuration of the graph suggests that indexes constructed for the four seasons may be even more revealing. If one were to do that, it would be found that surgical operations reach their highest level in summer, followed by spring and autumn in that order, with winter emerging as a season in which surgical activities are exceptionally low.

Hospital administrators are well aware that patient admissions have daily fluctuations. Admissions (all patients) are highest on Monday, followed closely by Tuesday. Wednesday, Thursday, and Sunday are days of moderate levels of admissions. The level of admissions drops somewhat on Friday and reaches its lowest point on Saturday. The daily pattern just described manifests itself in an exaggerated form if we focus on elective admissions alone.

Seasonal variations may be studied on an hourly basis too. For example, hospitals located in cities and metropolitan areas may experience hourly fluctuations in accident-related emergency arrivals: they tend to be high during morning and evening rush hours and low during the rest of the day.

Seasonal Indexes Defined

Seasonal indexes are quantitative measures of levels of activity. More specifically, the seasonal index for a specific month would show what is the expected level of activity during that month relative to the average level for the 12-month period (January through December). Seasonal indexes are expressed as proportions or percentages of the 12-month average. To bring out the meaning and significance of these proportions (or percentages), let us consider a simple example. Let us suppose that admissions during the 12-month period (January through December) total 1,200. The monthly average would then be 1,200 ÷ 12 = 100 admissions. If each month's share of admissions is 100, it means that admissions are distributed evenly over the months. In that case, the seasonal index for every month would be:

$$\frac{\text{Admissions during a specific month}}{\text{12-month average}} = \frac{100}{100} = 1.0000 \text{ (or 100.00)}$$

Let us now suppose that there are definite monthly ups and downs in the hospitalization of patients as shown in table 3-1. Here annual admissions total 1,200, yielding a monthly average of 100 admissions. The seasonal index for each month is obtained by dividing the actual admissions during each month by the 12-month average of 100 admissions. For example, the index for January is 105/100 = 1.05. Notice that the seasonal indexes for January, March, and December are 1.05, 1.00, and 0.91, respectively. What these figures mean is

Table 3-1
Monthly Admissions: A Hypothetical Example

	Jan.	Feb.	Mar.	Apr.	May	June	July	Aug.	Sept.	Oct.	Nov.	Dec.	Total	Average
Admissions	105	95	103	102	100	101	102	103	99	101	98	91	1,200	100
Seasonal Index	1.05	0.95	1.03	1.02	1.00	1.01	1.02	1.03	0.99	1.01	0.98	0.91	12.00	1.00

that January admissions run 5 percent above the 12-month average, March admissions are exactly equal to the 12-month average, and December admissions are only 91 percent of (or 9 percent below) the 12-month average.

The actual construction of seasonal indexes is somewhat more involved than the foregoing illustration. This is so because, as a rule, monthly data include not only seasonal variations, but variations caused by some other factors as well such as long-term trends, cyclical oscillations, and random disturbances. These factors are discussed in appendix I, and the construction methodology employed in this study is outlined in appendix II.

The reader is cautioned that the seasonal index for a given month, say, January, is constructed by averaging the fluctuations observed in several Januarys in the past. Therefore, the seasonal index constructed for January may not measure precisely the fluctuation that actually occurred in any particular January, say, January 1977, especially if some unusual episode such as a severe cold spell or an outbreak of influenza occurred during that month.[1] Nonetheless, the degree of fluctuation expressed by the index will be close enough to reality for all practical purposes.

Note

1. See chapter 5 for an explanation of the extent to which the actual value of an indicator for a specific month is likely to deviate from the value expressed by the seasonal index.

4

Practical Applications

The introductory chapter concluded with the statement that there are some limitations on the use of hospital indicators in their raw form. The purpose of this chapter is to amplify this statement and point out the advantages of de-seasonalizing raw values, that is, adjusting raw values with the aid of seasonal (monthly) indexes. It may be of interest to note that deseasonalizing time-series data is a standard procedure in use. For example, when governmental agencies release monthly statistics, the figures released are, in most cases, deseasonalized values. Here are the opening sentences of a Bureau of Labor Statistics periodical:

> This chartbook presents a comprehensive picture of current changes in prices, wages, costs, profits, and productivity in the U.S. economy. Most of the charts show *seasonally adjusted* or annual rates of change [emphasis added].[1]

The Significance of Seasonal Indexes

The meaning of seasonal indexes is briefly explained in chapter 3. We will now elaborate on this explanation and discuss the ways in which these indexes may be used with actual examples. It is important to note that all the examples given in this chapter are based on the seasonal indexes pertaining to the nation displayed in chapter 5. Those who plan to use the seasonal indexes for a segment of the hospital universe, such as a state, must use the appropriate regional indexes provided in tables 7-2 through 7-10.

Turning to figure 5-25, (p. 75) we find that the January index of adjusted expenses per inpatient day is 0.9528, while the December index is 1.0638. This means that adjusted expenses per inpatient day tend to be low in the month of January—about 95.28 percent of the annual average—and tend to be high in the month of December—about 106.38 percent of the annual average.

We can estimate what would have been the adjusted expenses per inpatient day in, say, January 1975 and December 1975, if admissions were uniform over the months. This can be done by simply dividing the raw values of January 1975 and December 1975 by the corresponding monthly indexes. The results, based on the National Hospital Panel Survey, are presented in table 4-1. Note that if we compute the rate of increase in adjusted expenses per inpatient day from January to December based on the deseasonalized values, we get a valid estimate,

Table 4–1
Adjusted Expenses per Impatient Day

Period	Raw Value[a]	Percent Change	Deseasonalized Value	Percent Change
Jan. 1975	$123.33	–	$123.33/0.9528 = $129.44	–
Dec. 1975	$158.51	28.53	$158.51/1.0638 = $149.00	15.11

[a]Source: "Hospital Indicators," *Hospitals,* April 16, 1975 and March 16, 1976. Reprinted with permission.

15.11 percent. Had we used the raw values, the result would have been a misleading estimate of rate of increase, 28.53 percent.

Let us consider another example. According to the National Hospital Panel Survey, the occupancy rate of community hospitals averaged 80.30 percent in February 1975 and 68.90 in December 1975. Turning to figure 5-16, we note that the February index of occupancy rate is 1.0609, and the December index is 0.9292. As before, we can estimate what would have been the occupancy rates of February 1975 and December 1975 if community hospitals experienced an even flow of patients. The relevant figures are shown in table 4–2.

If we base our calculations on the deseasonalized values, the absolute decline in occupancy rate during the 10-month period would be 75.69 - 74.15 = 1.54, or about one and a half percentage points. If we rely on the raw values, on the other hand, we get a potentially misleading figure, namely, 80.30 - 68.90 = 11.40 percentage points.

The process of dividing a raw value by the appropriate monthly index is called *deseasonalization,* and the resulting value is variously referred to as the *deseasonalized value,* the *seasonally adjusted value,* and the *value adjusted for seasonality.*

We will now attempt to indicate some specific areas of application of the monthly indexes reported in chapter 5 and table 7-1.

Table 4–2
Adult Occupancy Rate

Period	Raw Value[a]	Change in Percentage Points	Deseasonalized Value	Change in Percentage Points
Feb. 1975	80.30%	–	80.30%/1.0609 = 75.69%	–
Dec. 1975	68.90%	-11.40	68.90%/0.9292 = 74.15%	-1.54

[a]Source: "Hospital Indicators," *Hospitals,* May 16, 1975 and March 16, 1976. Reprinted with permission.

1. Deseasonalized Values are More Meaningful

Frequently, the American Hospital Association, allied health associations, and member hospitals are called upon to release the latest available figures on utilization, expenses, capacity utilization, and so on. For example, they may be called upon to release the latest figures on admissions, adjusted expenses per inpatient day, occupancy rates, and so on. What is traditionally done in these situations is to release the latest raw figures available. However, as we have seen already, raw monthly figures can be quite misleading. It is therefore suggested that the hospital system follow a practice similar to that adopted by governmental agencies. That is, release the latest figures in a deseasonalized form by dividing the raw figures by the appropriate monthly indexes. Of course, if raw figures are specifically asked for, they may be provided with a statement to the effect that they are subject to seasonal bias.

Perhaps another way of looking at deseasonalized values is as follows: Deseasonalization smoothes out aberrations in the monthly values of hospital indicators caused by seasonal fluctuations in the level of activity. It does not alter the annual totals or annual averages in any way. It simply redistributes the values evenly over the months. Table 4-3 bears this out. Notice that the annual average based on deseasonalized values ($137.80) is very close to the annual average based on raw values ($137.92). The slight discrepancy is due to the fact that the monthly indexes have been rounded off. In the case of absolute measures, such as total expenses, total patient days, etc., the annual totals obtained

Table 4-3
Adjusted Expenses per Inpatient Day, 1975

1 Month	2 Raw Value[a]	3 Seasonal Index	4 Deseasonalized Value (Col. 2 ÷ Col. 3)
January	$123.33	0.9528	$129.44
February	126.74	0.9760	129.86
March	128.56	0.9667	132.99
April	131.99	0.9856	133.92
May	135.69	0.9865	137.55
June	139.26	1.0244	135.94
July	141.20	1.0252	137.73
August	144.20	1.0165	141.86
September	141.96	1.0187	139.36
October	139.62	0.9879	141.33
November	144.03	0.9960	144.61
December	158.51	1.0638	149.00
Average	$137.92	1.0000	$137.80

[a]Source: "Hospital Indicators," *Hospitals,* various issues. Reprinted with permission.

by summing the raw values and deseasonalized values would, likewise, differ only by a rounding error.

2. Trend Analysis and Forecasting

The presence of seasonal ups and downs in the raw data obfuscates underlying trends, if any. If the raw data are deseasonalized and then plotted on a graph, the underlying trend can be better assessed. Figure 4-1 is an example in point. The solid line which represents raw figures on adult occupancy rate gives the erroneous impression that occupancy rate is declining sharply. The dotted line which represents deseasonalized figures provides an entirely different perspective—a perspective that accords with the true situation: occupancy rate remains around the 75 percent level.

It is almost mandatory that deseasonalized values be used to compute the percentage change of hospital indicators between any two time periods. Those who work with raw values can only compute 12-month percentage changes be-

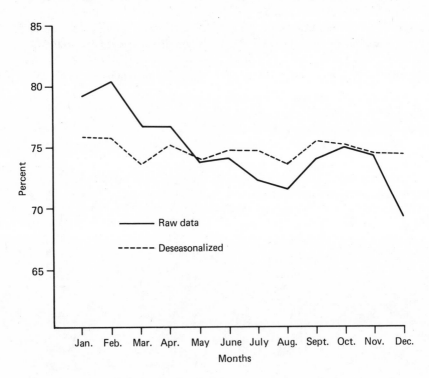

Figure 4-1. Adult Occupancy Rate, 1975

Table 4-4
Percentage Change in Adjusted Expense per Inpatient Day, 1975

| | | Percentage Change | |
| | | Based on | Based on Deseasonalized |
Time Period	Duration	Raw Values	Values
Sept.–Oct.	1 month	−1.6%	1.4%
Jan.–Apr.	3 months	7.0	3.5
Jan.–July	6 months	14.5	6.4
Jan.–Dec.	11 months	28.5	15.1

cause, in order to avoid seasonal bias, they must ensure that the initial and terminal months are the same. Examples are January 1975 to January 1976, July 1975 to July 1976, December 1975 to December 1976, and so on. Although this is a valid procedure, it is highly restrictive in that no other time period can be chosen. For example, if one has to ascertain percentage change during any two time periods where the initial and terminal months are different, raw figures produce misleading results. To illustrate, table 4-4 shows the percentage change in adjusted expenses per inpatient day during selected time periods in 1975. The values are taken from table 4-3. Notice that while the percentage changes computed from raw values are potentially misleading, the percentage changes computed from deseasonalized values are valid.

Deseasonalized values can be used effectively to make short- and intermediate-term forecasting. In what follows, we will illustrate a simple forecasting method—the graphic method. When state and metropolitan hospital associations and individual hospitals employ this method, they should use the data pertaining to their respective regions or institutions.

For short- and intermediate-range forecasting, we recommend the use of data pertaining to the latest 12-month period available. The selection of this time frame represents an optimum compromise between the stability inherent in past data and the sensitivity inherent in recent data.

For illustrative purposes, we will assume that the expense data available for the latest 12-month period pertain to December 1976 through November 1977. The first step involves deseasonalizing the raw data, as shown in table 4-5. Plot the deseasonalized values on graph paper, as shown in figure 4-2. Next, draw a trend line by visual inspection, as shown in the graph. Drawing trend lines by visual inspection is more of an art than anything else, although a rule of thumb is to ensure that about half the plot points are above the trend line and half below it. Having drawn the trend line, read off values as shown by the dotted lines in the graph. Turning to figure 4-2, projected total expenses for January 1978 will be about $4.73 billion. Of course, this value is in the deseasonalized

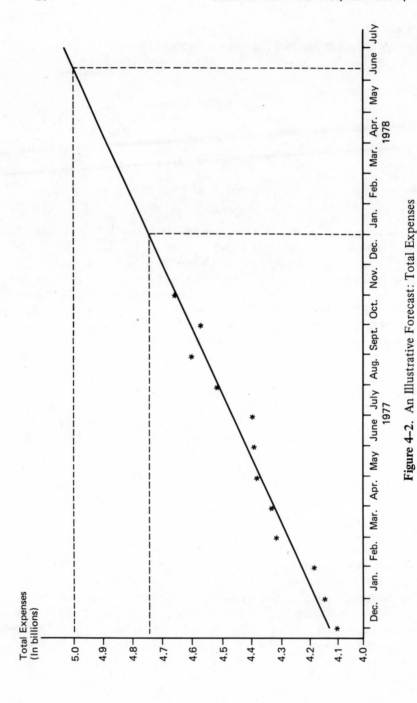

Figure 4-2. An Illustrative Forecast: Total Expenses

Table 4-5
Total Expenses, December 1976–November 1977
(billions of dollars)

Period	Raw Value[a]	Seasonal Index	Deseasonalized Value (Raw Value ÷ Seasonal Index)
1976 Dec.	$4.123	1.0073	$4.093
1977 Jan.	4.177	1.0103	4.134
Feb.	4.006	0.9611	4.168
Mar.	4.407	1.0245	4.302
Apr.	4.278	0.9921	4.312
May	4.387	1.0061	4.360
June	4.392	1.0040	4.375
July	4.448	1.0151	4.382
Aug.	4.561	1.0102	4.515
Sept.	4.516	0.9844	4.588
Oct.	4.583	1.0053	4.559
Nov.	4.552	0.9798	4.646

[a]Source: "Hospital Indicators," *Hospitals,* various issues. Reprinted with permission.

form. If one wishes to convert it back to the raw value, it should be multiplied by the appropriate seasonal index. For example, the raw value for January 1978 is (4.73 X 1.0103) = $4.78 billion.

If annual total expenses for a calendar year needs to be estimated, the following procedure is recommended. Read off the value corresponding to the midyear (June-July), and then multiply the value obtained by 12. Returning to figure 4-2, the value corresponding to June-July 1978 is $4.99 billion. Therefore, the projected total expenses for 1978 is (4.99 X 12) $59.88 billion. These projections are merely illustrative. They do not constitute the official projections of the American Hospital Association.[2]

3. Estimation of Annual Totals from Monthly Values

Instances may arise when annual totals of some measures have to be estimated from monthly data. Deseasonalized monthly values may then be used to make such an estimate. The example in table 4-6 illustrates the procedure.

Annual totals can be estimated by multiplying the deseasonalized value of any month by 12, as shown in column 5 of table 4-6. Notice that the annual totals estimated in this way are not far off the actual total, 2,991,000. Had we used the raw values, the results would have been quite unpredictable. For example, the annual total based on the raw data of April would have been 237,000

Table 4-6
Births, 1975

1	2	3	4	5
			Deseasonalized Births	*Estimated Annual Total*
	Births[a]	*Seasonal*	*(in 000s)*	*(in 000s)*
Month	*(in 000s)*	*Index*	*(Col. 2 ÷ Col. 3)*	*(Col. 4 × 12)*
Jan.	242	0.9803	247	2,964
Feb.	226	0.9175	246	2,952
Mar.	246	0.9949	247	2,964
Apr.	237	0.9374	253	3,036
May	246	0.9739	253	3,036
June	241	0.9710	248	2,976
July	262	1.0562	248	2,976
Aug.	269	1.0719	251	3,012
Sept.	271	1.0588	256	3,072
Oct.	258	1.0402	248	2,976
Nov.	238	0.9823	242	2,904
Dec.	255	1.0158	251	3,012
Total	2,991			

[a]Source: "Hospital Indicators," *Hospitals,* various issues. Reprinted with permission.

× 12 = 2,844,000, while the annual total based on the raw data of September would have been 271,000 × 12 = 3,252,000.

If an upward or downward trend is present, it is important to select the deseasonalized value of that month which is closest to the middle of the year in order to take account of the trend factor. For example, if the deseasonalized value of June or July is available, one of these or, preferably, an average of these should be multiplied by 12 to estimate the annual total.

4. Assessment of Facilities and Resource Needs

The seasonal indexes of adult occupancy rate, average daily census, and adjusted patient days show periods of peaks and troughs in the overall demand facing hospitals. This knowledge is helpful to administrators in planning for facilities and resources in tune with anticipated month to month variations in demand. Also, the seasonal indexes of births, newborn occupancy rates, surgical operations, and outpatient visits reveal that these activities have peaks and troughs of their own. This knowledge also is helpful in planning for specialized facilities and resources.

5. Financial Management

A hospital's financial position may be affected by seasonality in the demand for its services. This is particularly so in regard to short-term indicators of financial position, such as current assets, current liabilities, operating margin, current ratio, and "quick" ratio.

6. Cost Accounting

Accounting departments may find it necessary to recognize seasonal variation when they compute unit costs if these costs are to be used for purposes of control. If seasonal variation is not recognized, unit costs during seasonally slack periods may include, for example, unavoidable idle time on facilities, machines, and equipment.

7. Interrelationship between Hospital Indicators

Practically every hospital indicator reported in this study is related to or influenced by one or several other indicators in some form or another.[3] A better understanding of these relations and influences is helpful in two ways: First, it enhances the ability of hospital management to bring about desired changes in the operating characteristics of hospitals. Second, it enables hospital management to see more clearly the impact of their decisions on hospital indicators. A useful feature of seasonal indexes is that they bring relations and influences into sharper focus. Thus, we see, for example, the following:

Admissions, patient days, and total revenue fluctuate in unison. Average daily census and adult occupancy follow the same basic pattern.

Adjusted expenses per inpatient day—a key statistic of the hospital industry— fluctuates in a direction opposite to the preceding group of indicators.

There is an almost perfect correlation between the fluctuations of adjusted patient days and total revenue.

Adult length of stay—an important determinant of expenses per admission— is generally longer in the winter season.

Surgical operations and outpatient visits tend to fluctuate in concert.

The seasonal pattern of newborn utilization indicators is different from that of adult utilization indicators.

If we compare the graph of adult occupancy rate (figure 5-16) with those of newborn occupancy rate (figure 5-17) and outpatient visits (figure 5-5), an interesting picture emerges: newborn and outpatient activities have peaks when adult patient activity has troughs. Thus the presence of newborn nurseries and outpatient departments seems to impart the type of stability one associates with product diversification. It moderates extreme fluctuations in the level of activity, and thereby enhances the ability of hospitals to achieve a better match between facilities and resources, on the one hand, and the demand for services, on the other.

Adult occupancy rate runs below average during summer and drops sharply in December (figure 5-16), a month when surgical operations drop to a level not reached by any other indicator (figure 5-19). Hospital managers can moderate the adverse consequences of excess capacity if they capitalize on the known preferences of consumers and schedule more elective surgery and associated admissions in summer. Since it may not be easy to schedule more elective surgery in December, the introduction of techniques such as the "5-day medical-surgical unit" discussed in chapter 5 may be considered.

Notes

1. U.S. Department of Labor, Bureau of Labor Statistics, *Chartbook on Prices, Wages, and Productivity*, May 1977, Washington, p. 1.

2. Those who are statistically inclined may fit the trend line by the method of least squares. As a matter of interest, such a trend line was derived, and it took the following form:

$$TE = 4.04812 + 0.0494T$$

where *TE* is projected total expenses, and *T* is the time unit expressed in months, (that is, December 1976 = 1, January 1977 = 2, and so on). If we use this trend equation, total expenses for January 1978 and June-July 1978 will be:

January 1978 = 4.04812 + 0.04943 (14) = \$4.74 billion

June-July 1978 = 4.04812 + 0.04943 (19.5) = \$5.01 billion

Notice that these values are very close to \$4.73 billion and \$4.99 billion projected earlier using the graphic method.

If desired, one may also derive the equation defining the trend line drawn in figure 4-2. This can be done by selecting any two points on the trend line, reading off the coordinates, and applying the following formula:

$$TE = E_1 + \frac{E_2 - E_1}{T_2 - T_1}(T - T_1)$$

We have selected two points on the trend line corresponding to January 1977 and April 1978 which yielded the following values:

$$TE = 4.16 + \frac{4.87 - 4.16}{17 - 2}(T - 2)$$

which resulted in the following trend equation:

$$TE = 4.06533 + 0.04733T$$

3. A glossary of the more important relationships is provided at the end of this book.

5 National Indexes

In this chapter we will examine, in some detail, the seasonality of hospital statistics pertaining to the nation as a whole.

Taxonomy of Hospital Indicators

There are no hard and fast rules as to how hospital indicators should be classified. Much depends on the purpose at hand. The classification scheme adopted in this study is as follows:

Adult Utilization Measures

Inpatient days
Adjusted patient days
Admissions
Adjusted admissions
Outpatient visits
Adult length of stay

Newborn Utilization Measures

Births
Newborn days
Newborn length of stay

Utilization Measures: 65 and over age group

Admissions: age 65 and over
Inpatient days: age 65 and over
Length of stay: age 65 and over

Capacity Measures

Beds
Adult daily census
Adult occupancy rate
Newborn Occupancy rate

Surgical Operations

Revenue Measures

Total revenue
Revenue per adjusted patient day
Revenue per adjusted admission

Expense Measures

Total expenses
Adjusted expenses per inpatient day
Adjusted expenses per admission

Presentation Format

A page has been devoted to each hospital indicator. This page includes a graph of the monthly indexes pertaining to the indicator, accompanied by a table that lists actual index values. Displayed on the graph is a measure of amplitude (*MA*). This is the standard deviation (variability) of index values pertaining to the months of January through December. It is a measure of amplitude in the sense that greater month-to-month fluctuations will produce larger *MA* values, and vice versa. The *MA* values provide a convenient means of comparing the degree of monthly fluctuations of various hospital indicators. For example, surgical operations (figure 5-19) has an *MA* value of 0.055, signifying a high degree of monthly fluctuations, while beds (figure 5-14) has an *MA* value of 0.002, signifying a low degree of monthly fluctuations.

The index values are displayed above the dotted line in the table. Turning to figure 5-3, for example, we see that the January index of admissions is 1.0490. This means that admissions in January are higher than the annual average by 4.9 percent. The February index, on the other hand, is 0.9571. This means that admissions in February are only 95.71 percent of the annual average or, what is the same thing, 4.29 percent (1 – 0.9571 = 0.0429, or 4.29 percent) less than the annual average.

The monthly indexes are presented in ratio form. The deseasonalized value of a hospital indicator pertaining to any specific month, such as January 1977, February 1977, and so on, can be obtained by dividing the raw values of the indicator by the corresponding monthly indexes. To illustrate, let us use the January and February indexes of admissions given in figure 5-3. According to the National Hospital Panel Survey, raw values of admisssions in January 1977 and February 1977 were 3,042,000 and 2,817,000, respectively.[1] Therefore, the seasonally adjusted admissions for January 1977 and February are 3,042,000 ÷ 1.0490 = 2,900,000 and 2,817,000 ÷ 0.9571 = 2,943,000, respectively.

An additional statistic—95 percent confidence interval—is provided below each monthly index. This value provides a measure of the temporal stability or constancy of the monthly index, that is, how much the index pertaining to a month is likely to vary from year to year. The smaller this value, the greater the stability, and vice versa.[2] For example, in figure 5-1, a value of 0.0163 is given below the January index of 1.0666. This means that the January index of each year would lie, 95 percent of the time, between the lower bound of 1.0503 (that is, 1.0666 - 0.0163) and the upper bound of 1.0829 (that is, 1.0666 + 0.0163).

Examination of the confidence intervals reveals that certain hospital indicators have greater temporal stability than others. For example, the confidence intervals shown against inpatient days, adjusted patient days, adult daily census, beds, adult occupancy rate, total expenses, and adjusted expenses per inpatient day are rather narrow—slightly over 1 percent—indicating a high degree of temporal stability. The confidence intervals associated with surgical operations and outpatient visits, on the other hand, are much broader—4 to 5 percent— indicating a low degree of temporal stability. The confidence intervals associated with the remaining hospital indicators lie somewhere between these extremes.

The Leap-Year Effect

To capture the effect of leap year precisely, it would have been necessary to construct two sets of indexes, one for leap years and another for standard years. A more convenient—albeit less precise—alternative is to estimate the effect of leap year on the February indexes.

Column 2 of table 5-1 shows what the index values of February would have been if the data pertaining entirely to leap years were used for the construction of February indexes. Column 3 shows the differences between these indexes and the corresponding indexes reported in this book. As one might expect, the effect of an additional day in February is a slight increase in all thirteen aggregate (volumetric) indicators. However, leap year causes a slight decline in the index values pertaining to revenue per adjusted patient day and adjusted expenses per inpatient day. Although the reason for this decline may not be all that obvious, an answer could be found in the change that has occurred in adult length of stay. Leap year causes an increase in length of stay, and as we have seen (chapter 1), the lengthier the stay, the lower the per diem expenses and the revenue charged to cover the expenses. Also note that leap year causes a slight increase in revenue per adjusted admission and adjusted expenses per admission. These results are consistent with the relationships depicted in figure 5-6.

A priori, one would have expected no change or possibly a slight decline in capacity utilization measures. As it turns out, leap year causes a very slight increase in adult daily census and occupancy rate. Newborn occupancy rate does show a very slight decline, however. It should be noted that the differences

Table 5-1
The Leap-Year Effect on February Indexes: National

Indicator	1 Seasonal Index	2 Seasonal Index Based on Leap Years Alone	3 Difference (Col. 2- Col. 1)
Inpatient days	0.9881	1.0053	0.0172
Admissions	0.9571	0.9668	0.0097
Adjusted admissions	0.9538	0.9611	0.0073
Adjusted patient days	0.9840	1.0011	0.0171
Adult length of stay	1.0315	1.0391	0.0076
Adult daily census	1.0635	1.0663	0.0028
Beds	1.0025	1.0033	0.0008
Occupancy rate	1.0609	1.0626	0.0017
Births	0.9175	0.9302	0.0127
Newborn days	0.9267	0.9375	0.0108
Newborn length of stay	1.0115	1.0236	0.0121
Newborn occupancy rate	0.9988	0.9959	-0.0029
Admissions: age 65 and over	0.9540	0.9743	0.0203
Inpatient days: age 65 and over	0.9709	0.9993	0.0284
Length of stay: age 65 and over	1.0155	1.0279	0.0124
Surgical operations	0.9470	0.9628	0.0158
Outpatient visits	0.9328	0.9525	0.0197
Total revenue	0.9759	0.9922	0.0163
Revenue per adjusted patient day	0.9908	0.9897	-0.0011
Revenue per adjusted admission	1.0214	1.0217	0.0003
Total expenses	0.9611	0.9721	0.0110
Adjusted expenses per Inpatient day	0.9760	0.9694	-0.0066
Adjusted expenses per admission	1.0066	1.0113	0.0047

shown in column 3 of table 5-1 would have been somewhat more pronounced if two sets of indexes—one based exclusively on standard years and another based exclusively on leap years—were constructed.

Adult Utilization Measures

Inpatient Days and Adjusted Patient Days

Inpatient days and adjusted patient days are the most popular measures of hospital output. The latter, of course, is the more adequate measure of output in that it includes outpatient visits as well. Turning to figure 5-1, we see that inpatient days tend to be high during the early part of the year and low during the later part. It is obvious that climatic conditions influence hospitalization

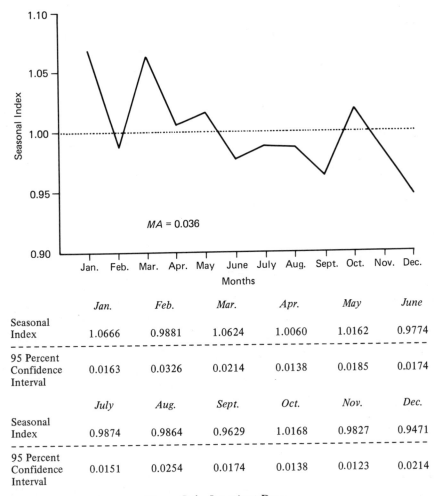

	Jan.	Feb.	Mar.	Apr.	May	June
Seasonal Index	1.0666	0.9881	1.0624	1.0060	1.0162	0.9774
95 Percent Confidence Interval	0.0163	0.0326	0.0214	0.0138	0.0185	0.0174
	July	Aug.	Sept.	Oct.	Nov.	Dec.
Seasonal Index	0.9874	0.9864	0.9629	1.0168	0.9827	0.9471
95 Percent Confidence Interval	0.0151	0.0254	0.0174	0.0138	0.0123	0.0214

Figure 5–1. Inpatient Days

rates. More people are hospitalized during the winter season than in spring or summer.

Monthly fluctuations are substantial, reaching a high of 1.0666 (or 6.66 percent above average) in January reflecting the combined effect of inclement weather and the pent-up demand of December. The index values are consistently below average during the summer months of June, July, August, and September. The unusually low index value for December (0.9471, or 5.29 percent below average) is a characteristic feature of hospital utilization. It is a month in which consumers, doctors, and hospital personnel would rather be someplace else than in the hospital.

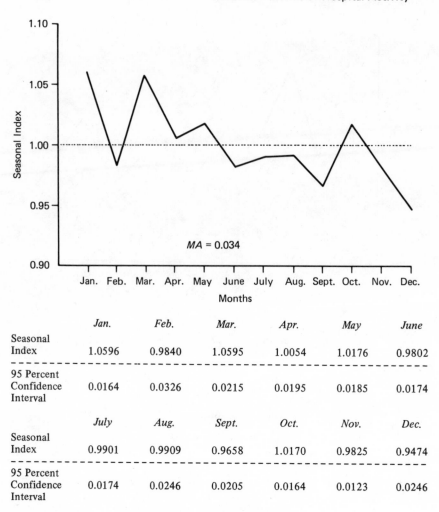

	Jan.	Feb.	Mar.	Apr.	May	June
Seasonal Index	1.0596	0.9840	1.0595	1.0054	1.0176	0.9802
95 Percent Confidence Interval	0.0164	0.0326	0.0215	0.0195	0.0185	0.0174
	July	Aug.	Sept.	Oct.	Nov.	Dec.
Seasonal Index	0.9901	0.9909	0.9658	1.0170	0.9825	0.9474
95 Percent Confidence Interval	0.0174	0.0246	0.0205	0.0164	0.0123	0.0246

Figure 5-2. Adjusted Patient Days

The graph of adjusted patient days (figure 5-2) looks like the "mirror image" of the one drawn for patient days (figure 5-1). But there is a significant difference. The amplitude of monthly fluctuations is less severe for adjusted patient days than it is for inpatient days. This is indicated by the measure of amplitude (*MA*), which is only 0.034 for adjusted patient days as opposed to 0.036 for inpatient days. Why is this so? Outpatient visits have a seasonal pattern that runs counter to the seasonal pattern of inpatient days (see figure 5-5). Thus outpatient care serves as a stabilizing force—it moderates monthly fluctuations in hospital activity.

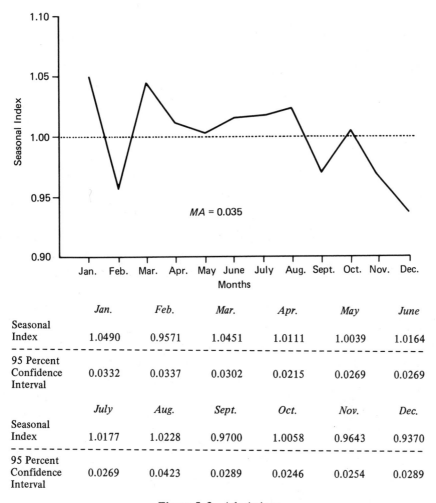

	Jan.	Feb.	Mar.	Apr.	May	June
Seasonal Index	1.0490	0.9571	1.0451	1.0111	1.0039	1.0164
95 Percent Confidence Interval	0.0332	0.0337	0.0302	0.0215	0.0269	0.0269

	July	Aug.	Sept.	Oct.	Nov.	Dec.
Seasonal Index	1.0177	1.0228	0.9700	1.0058	0.9643	0.9370
95 Percent Confidence Interval	0.0269	0.0423	0.0289	0.0246	0.0254	0.0289

Figure 5-3. Admissions

Admissions and Adjusted Admissions

Admissions (figure 5-3) and its synonyms, such as discharges, cases, and epi-sodes, represent an alternative measure of hospital output. Adjusted admissions (figure 5-4) is a composite of admissions and outpatient visits converted to equivalent admission units.

There are some similarities between the seasonal patterns of admissions and inpatient days, but the differences are noteworthy. The February and December dips of admissions are more severe than that of inpatient days. Unlike inpatient

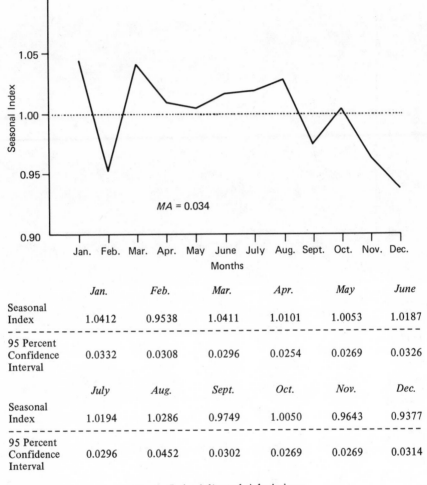

	Jan.	Feb.	Mar.	Apr.	May	June
Seasonal Index	1.0412	0.9538	1.0411	1.0101	1.0053	1.0187
95 Percent Confidence Interval	0.0332	0.0308	0.0296	0.0254	0.0269	0.0326

	July	Aug.	Sept.	Oct.	Nov.	Dec.
Seasonal Index	1.0194	1.0286	0.9749	1.0050	0.9643	0.9377
95 Percent Confidence Interval	0.0296	0.0452	0.0302	0.0269	0.0269	0.0314

Figure 5-4. Adjusted Admissions

days, admissions are above average during the summer months. This paradox may be explained in terms of variations in length of stay. Turning to figure 5-7, we note that length of stay tends to be short in the summer months. Since inpatient days, by definition, equals admissions times length of stay, the shorter length of stay during the summer months causes inpatient days to fall below average.

The seasonal pattern of adjusted admissions is basically the same as that of admissions. The only observable difference is that the indexes of adjusted admissions pertaining to summer months are slightly higher than the corresponding indexes of admissions.

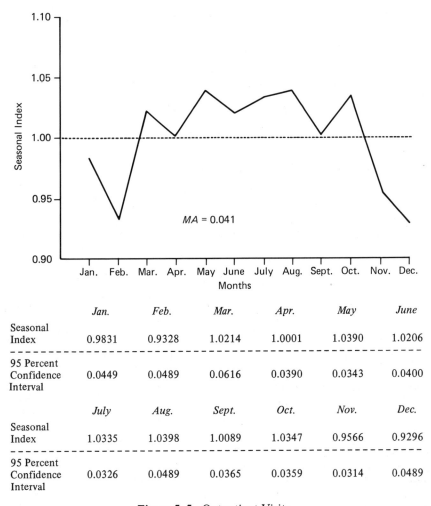

	Jan.	Feb.	Mar.	Apr.	May	June
Seasonal Index	0.9831	0.9328	1.0214	1.0001	1.0390	1.0206
95 Percent Confidence Interval	0.0449	0.0489	0.0616	0.0390	0.0343	0.0400

	July	Aug.	Sept.	Oct.	Nov.	Dec.
Seasonal Index	1.0335	1.0398	1.0089	1.0347	0.9566	0.9296
95 Percent Confidence Interval	0.0326	0.0489	0.0365	0.0359	0.0314	0.0489

Figure 5-5. Outpatient Visits

Outpatient Visits

We have already alluded to the rapid growth of outpatient visits during the past 14 years (figure 2-1). This trend is likely to continue and may even accelerate because of the growing emphasis on outpatient care as a cost-containment device. For example, the Carter administration's Hospital Cost Containment Bill (H.R. 6575/S. 1391) excludes from control revenue derived from outpatient services and thereby seeks to encourage the substitution of outpatient care, wherever possible, for inpatient care.

The seasonality of Outpatient Visits (figure 5-5) exhibits several noteworthy features. First, month-to-month fluctuations in the level of outpatient activity are much greater than any indicator considered so far. For example, outpatient visits have an *MA* value of 0.041 compared with 0.035 for admissions and 0.036 for inpatient days. Second, outpatient visits are high during spring and summer—periods when inpatient days are low. A possible explanation is the higher incidences of accidents and crimes during summer and spring, when people generally spend more time outdoors. Finally, there are striking similarities between the seasonal patterns of outpatient visits and surgical operations (see figure 5-19).

Adult Length of Stay

Adult length of stay, or length of stay, for short, is an important and revealing statistic in many ways. Length of stay is a determinant of inhospital utilization in that inpatient days equals admissions times length of stay. It is also indicative of case severity and the age of the patient. The more severe the case and the older the patient, the lengthier generally will be his or her stay in the hospital.

We have already touched on the inverse relationship between length of stay and per diem expenses (see chapter 1). To provide a more revealing picture of the interrelationship between length of stay, on the one hand, and various expense measures, on the other, we have constructed figure 5-6 based on the 1966-67 charge data reported by the Social Security Administration.[3] The three expense measures plotted on the graph are:

    EPD: Expenses per inpatient day

    EPA: Expenses per admission

    ESDA: Expenses specific to each day after admission. That is, expenses incurred on the first day after admisssion, the second day after admission, and so on.

Notice that *ESDA* is a maximum ($110) on the first day of admission. As the patient stays longer, *ESDA* decreases sharply at first and slowly later on. By the seventh or eighth day of admission, *ESDA* reaches its lowest point ($50) and levels off. This phenomenon has important implications for *EPD* and *EPA*.

Consider, for instance, a hospitalization episode lasting 2 days. The *EPD* for this episode is very high ($98), whereas the *EPA* is very low ($197). Contrast this with the corresponding expense statistics pertaining to a hospitalization episode lasting 16 days: *EPD* = $58 and *EPA* = $936. In fact, if we extend figure 5-6 to cover lengthier stays, *EPD* would continue to fall until it approaches *ESDA*. For a hospitalization episode lasting 50 days, for example, the *EPD* would be only $53, while *EPA* would be a whopping $2,636. We can now make

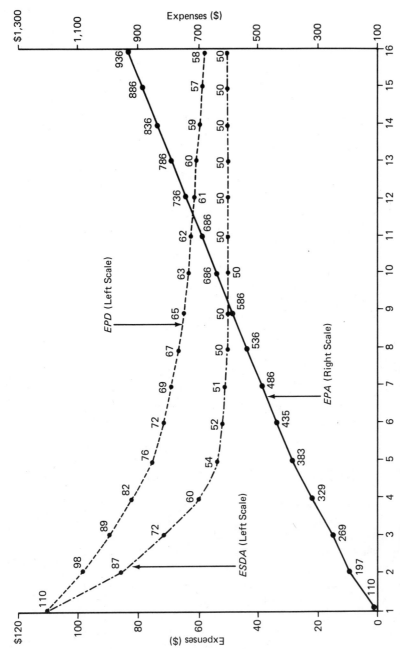

Figure 5-6. Interrelationship between Length of Stay and Three Expense Measures

Source: U.S. Dept. of HEW, S.S.A., *Selected Charge Pattern in Short-Stay Hospitals under Medicare*, Prepared in the Division of Health Insurance Studies, Office of Research and Statistics, No. HI-31, Sept. 30, 1971, Chart B.

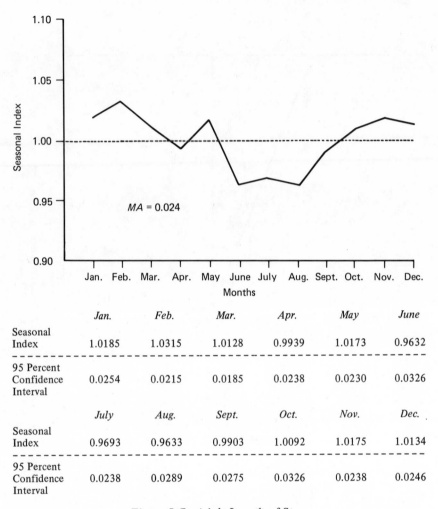

	Jan.	*Feb.*	*Mar.*	*Apr.*	*May*	*June*
Seasonal Index	1.0185	1.0315	1.0128	0.9939	1.0173	0.9632
95 Percent Confidence Interval	0.0254	0.0215	0.0185	0.0238	0.0230	0.0326

	July	*Aug.*	*Sept.*	*Oct.*	*Nov.*	*Dec.*
Seasonal Index	0.9693	0.9633	0.9903	1.0092	1.0175	1.0134
95 Percent Confidence Interval	0.0238	0.0289	0.0275	0.0326	0.0238	0.0246

Figure 5-7. Adult Length of Stay

two general statements. The shorter the length of stay, the higher the *EPD* and the lower the *EPA*. Conversely, the lengthier the stay, the lower the *EPD* and the higher the *EPA*.

The seasonal pattern of adult length of stay is displayed in figure 5-7. Length of stay is shortest during the summer months and longest during the winter months. One possible explanation is the higher proportion of patients aged 65 and over during the winter months (see figure 5-11). Aged patients, who represent roughly 25 percent of the total patient population, had an average length of stay of 10.7 days in 1977 as opposed to 7.2 days for all adult patients.

Another possible reason for seasonal variation in adult length of stay is the correlation between the occurrence of certain diseases and weather conditions.

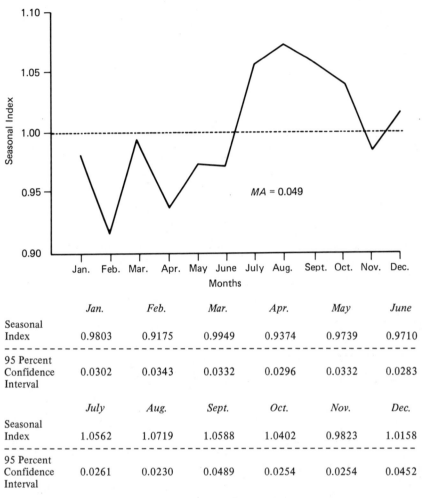

	Jan.	*Feb.*	*Mar.*	*Apr.*	*May*	*June*
Seasonal Index	0.9803	0.9175	0.9949	0.9374	0.9739	0.9710
95 Percent Confidence Interval	0.0302	0.0343	0.0332	0.0296	0.0332	0.0283

	July	*Aug.*	*Sept.*	*Oct.*	*Nov.*	*Dec.*
Seasonal Index	1.0562	1.0719	1.0588	1.0402	0.9823	1.0158
95 Percent Confidence Interval	0.0261	0.0230	0.0489	0.0254	0.0254	0.0452

Figure 5-8. Births

For example, coronary heart diseases, which entail lengthier stays, occur more frequently when the temperature falls below 40°F with or without snowfall.[4]

Newborn Utilization Measures

Births

Births (figure 5-8) display a high degree of seasonality. The large MA value (0.049) and the fact that indexes range from a high of 1.0719 (or 7.19 percent above average) to a low of 0.9175 (or 8.25 percent below average) amply illus-

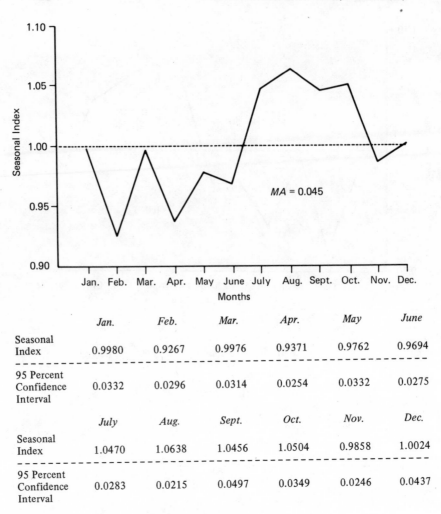

	Jan.	Feb.	Mar.	Apr.	May	June
Seasonal Index	0.9980	0.9267	0.9976	0.9371	0.9762	0.9694
95 Percent Confidence Interval	0.0332	0.0296	0.0314	0.0254	0.0332	0.0275
	July	Aug.	Sept.	Oct.	Nov.	Dec.
Seasonal Index	1.0470	1.0638	1.0456	1.0504	0.9858	1.0024
95 Percent Confidence Interval	0.0283	0.0215	0.0497	0.0349	0.0246	0.0437

Figure 5-9. Newborn Days

trate the breadth of seasonality. Peaking in August, births remain high in the fall. Spring months are characterized by exceptionally low birth rates. We have already referred to the link between climatic conditions and conception rates (chapter 1). According to Pasamanick et al., high temperatures may reduce sexual activity and adversely affect the viability of sperm, thereby reducing conception rates.[5] Chang et al. pointed out that female fertility is also affected by high temperatures, which increase the incidence of amenorrhea.[6] Since the summer season falls roughly between June and September, births are low in spring, which arrives roughly 9 months after summer.

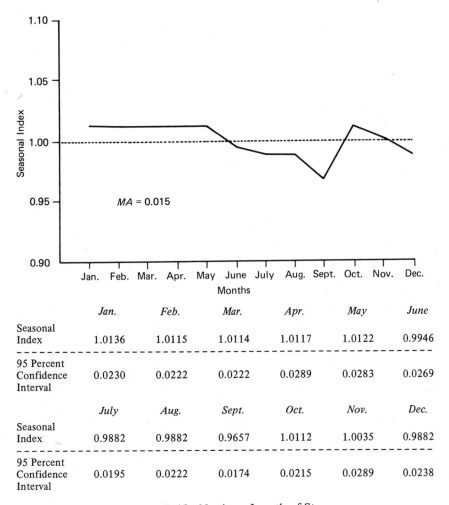

	Jan.	Feb.	Mar.	Apr.	May	June
Seasonal Index	1.0136	1.0115	1.0114	1.0117	1.0122	0.9946
95 Percent Confidence Interval	0.0230	0.0222	0.0222	0.0289	0.0283	0.0269

	July	Aug.	Sept.	Oct.	Nov.	Dec.
Seasonal Index	0.9882	0.9882	0.9657	1.0112	1.0035	0.9882
95 Percent Confidence Interval	0.0195	0.0222	0.0174	0.0215	0.0289	0.0238

Figure 5-10. Newborn Length of Stay

Newborn Days

The seasonal pattern of newborn days (figure 5-9) is almost identical with that of births. The only discernible difference is the slight drop in newborn days during September. This may be explained in terms of a similar drop of newborn length of stay during September (see figure 5-10).

Newborn Length of Stay

Monthly fluctuations in newborn length of stay (figure 5-10) are of low magnitude (MA = 0.015). From January to May, the indexes run slightly above average and drop below average during those months when births are high. The unusual drop in September and the fact that there is, generally speaking, an inverse relationship between newborn length of stay and birth rates lead one to infer that hospitals respond to increased demand for bassinets by faster turnover rates.[7]

Utilization Measures: 65 and Over Age Group

The adult utilization statistics presented in the preceding section include the data pertaining to the 65 and over age group. Nonetheless, this age group merits separate treatment for a number of reasons. This country has an aging population. The percent of U.S. population aged 65 and over, which stood at 9.8 in 1970, rose to 10.5 in 1975. It is estimated that by 1985, this age group will constitute 11.5 percent of the population.[8] Furthermore, the age distribution of the elderly population is gradually shifting to the right, with more people in the over-75 age group.

The level and pattern of hospital utilization by the elderly differ in certain aspects from those of the rest of the population. For example, on the average, a person aged 65 and over uses 4½ times as much hospital care and, once hospitalized, stays about 4 days more than a person under 65. In addition, there are also certain differences with respect to the seasonality of hospital utilization of the elderly. These differences are likely to be accentuated in the years ahead as the age distribution of the elderly continues to shift to the right. This section will examine similarities as well as differences, keeping in mind the fact that the inclusion of the data pertaining to the elderly in the adult utilization statistics has the effect of overstating similarities and understating differences.

Admissions: Age 65 and Over

In an overall sense, the seasonal pattern of admissions of this age group (figure 5-11) is similar to that of the adult population as a whole. But the following differences are noteworthy. The January upsurge is greater for this age group, running 7 percent above average as opposed to 5 percent for the adult population as a whole. Admissions in summer generally run below average, and the December slump is much less precipitous for this age group. It would appear that the 65 and over age group is more susceptible to the effects of cold and snowfall associated with winter than the younger populations.

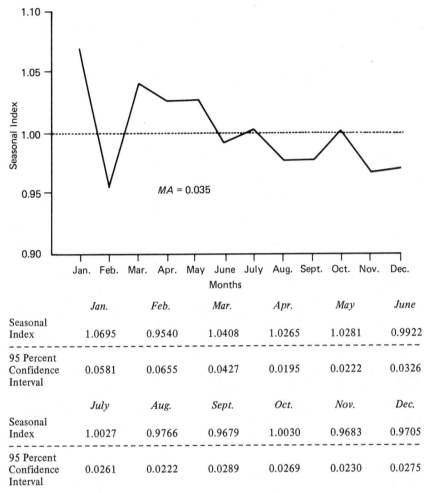

	Jan.	Feb.	Mar.	Apr.	May	June
Seasonal Index	1.0695	0.9540	1.0408	1.0265	1.0281	0.9922
95 Percent Confidence Interval	0.0581	0.0655	0.0427	0.0195	0.0222	0.0326
	July	Aug.	Sept.	Oct.	Nov.	Dec.
Seasonal Index	1.0027	0.9766	0.9679	1.0030	0.9683	0.9705
95 Percent Confidence Interval	0.0261	0.0222	0.0289	0.0269	0.0230	0.0275

Figure 5–11. Admissions: Age 65 and Over

Inpatient Days: Age 65 and Over

As in the case of admissions, the differential effects of winter are clearly in evidence from a comparison between the seasonal patterns of this age group and the adult population as a whole (figure 5–12). January inpatient days run 7.1 percent above average and December inpatient days are very close to the average as opposed to 6.7 percent above average and 5.3 percent below average, respectively, for the adult population as a whole.

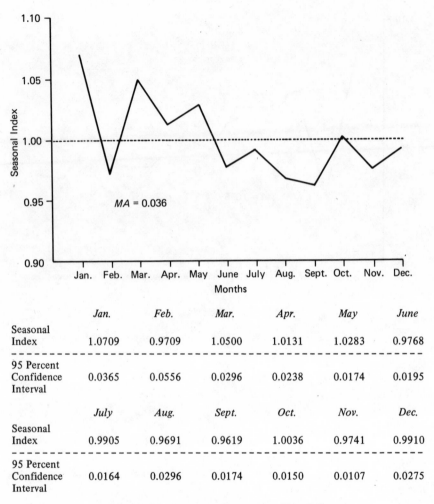

	Jan.	Feb.	Mar.	Apr.	May	June
Seasonal Index	1.0709	0.9709	1.0500	1.0131	1.0283	0.9768
95 Percent Confidence Interval	0.0365	0.0556	0.0296	0.0238	0.0174	0.0195

	July	Aug.	Sept.	Oct.	Nov.	Dec.
Seasonal Index	0.9905	0.9691	0.9619	1.0036	0.9741	0.9910
95 Percent Confidence Interval	0.0164	0.0296	0.0174	0.0150	0.0107	0.0275

Figure 5-12. Inpatient Days: Age 65 and Over

Length of Stay: Age 65 and Over

The length of stay of this age group and the adult population as a whole tends to be high in winter and low in summer (figure 5-13). But the similarity ends here. The length of stay of the elderly exhibits much less month-to-month variation (MA = 0.012) compared with that of adult population as a whole (MA = 0.024).

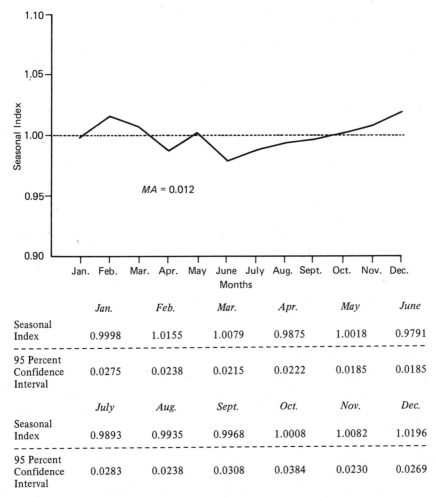

	Jan.	Feb.	Mar.	Apr.	May	June
Seasonal Index	0.9998	1.0155	1.0079	0.9875	1.0018	0.9791
95 Percent Confidence Interval	0.0275	0.0238	0.0215	0.0222	0.0185	0.0185

	July	Aug.	Sept.	Oct.	Nov.	Dec.
Seasonal Index	0.9893	0.9935	0.9968	1.0008	1.0082	1.0196
95 Percent Confidence Interval	0.0283	0.0238	0.0308	0.0384	0.0230	0.0269

Figure 5-13. Length of Stay: Age 65 and Over

Capacity Measures

Excess Capacity in the Hospital Industry

The number of adult and pediatric beds set up and staffed for use constitutes the overall measure of bed capacity in the hospital industry. *Excess capacity,* that is, the number or percentage of beds that remains unutilized, has become the focus of interest and polemics in recent times. In a report released in 1976, the Institute of Medicine raised the specter of "excess capacity" or "overbedding" as a major cause of escalating hospital costs.[9] The National Guidelines for Health Planning, contained in the National Health Planning Act (P.L. 93-641), set an occupancy rate of 80 percent (or an excess capacity of 20 percent) as the optimum level for all hospitals across the country.[10] Since current occupancy rate runs around 75 percent, the inference is that excess capacity is pervasive in the hospital industry.

The argument that excess capacity contributes to cost increase has a sound theoretical basis, and minimization of excess capacity to the furthest extent possible ought to be the goal of all private firms operating for a profit. However, in applying this principle to the hospital industry, the special circumstances surrounding the operation of hospitals should not be ignored. We have already indicated that if a hospital pursues this principle too far, its ability to meet community demands promptly will be compromised (chapter 1).

It may well be that excess capacity over and above what one may regard as reasonable does exist in certain institutions and/or geographic areas. But setting a single occupancy rate (80 percent) across the baord as the optimum can only be characterized as a "meat ax" approach to a complex problem.[11]

The Concept of Protection Level

A rational approach to capacity utilization by hospitals must involve the concept of *protection level,* that is, the ability of hospitals to meet community demand for hospital care adequately and expeditiously. If a hospital is operating at a protection level of, say, 95 percent, what is implied is that this hospital has the ability to admit, without delay, those who seek hospitalization 95 percent of the time. Putting it differently, the hospital in question is willing to tolerate an "overfill" or "turnaway" rate of 1 day in 20. The important point is that the protection level of a hospital hinges critically upon its bedside.

Protection Level and Hospital Size

The proposition that a given occupancy rate has different import to hospitals of varying sizes can be demonstrated intuitively and by statistical theory. Consider a ten-bed hospital maintaining an occupancy rate of 80 percent. It has only two empty beds to deal with any contingency that might arise. In contrast, a 1000-bed hospital maintaining the same occupancy rate has a cushion of 200 empty beds.

It is also possible to determine statistically the excess capacity required to maintain a given protection level.[12] These are shown in table 5-2 for selected

Table 5-2
Required Excess Capacity to Ensure a Protection Level of 95 Percent (or a Turnaway Rate of 1 Day in 20)

Bedsize	Average Daily Census	Required Excess Capacity		Corresponding Occupancy Rate
		In Beds	In Percentages	
10	5	5	50	50%
15	9	6	40	60
20	13	7	35	65
25	17	8	32	68
50	39	11	22	78
100	84	16	16	84
1,000	950	50	5	95

Table 5-3
Occupancy Rate: Community Hospitals, 1976

Bed Size	Occupancy Rate
6–24	45.7%
25–49	54.8
50–99	63.1
100–199	70.5
200–299	76.5
300–399	79.0
400–499	80.3
500+	80.9

Source: American Hospital Association, *Hospital Statistics,* 1977 ed., Table 3. Reprinted with permission.

bed sizes. Notice that as we move from small to large bed sizes, hospitals are able to meet the 95 percent protection criterion at higher and higher occupancy rates. It is because of the innate ability of larger hospitals to maintain higher occupancy rates that one finds a strong positive correlation between bed size and occupancy rate (see table 5-3).

The Assumption of Bed Interchangeability

We have seen that hospitals are, in reality, multiproduct firms providing a wide variety of services for the specialized needs of patients (chapter 1). Therefore, it is no surprise that the total bed complement of a modern hospital consists of general medical-surgical beds plus beds set up in several specialized units. Some examples of specialized units are:

Pediatric unit

Obstetric unit

Intensive care unit

Neonatal intensive care unit

Psychiatric unit

Rehabilitation unit

T.B. and other respiratory diseases unit

Alcoholism/chemical dependency unit

Burn care unit

The beds set up in the medical-surgical unit and each of the specialized units are, generally, not interchangeable. For example, a patient arriving for delivery must be housed in the obstetric unit.

Table 5–2 is based on the total bed capacity of hospitals and therefore assumes implicitly that all beds are interchangeable. Since this assumption is unrealistic, it is necessary to explore what the situation would be if the beds set up in each distinct unit are not interchangeable.

Let us assume that a 100-bed hospital is organized as follows: medical-surgical units, 50 beds; pediatric unit, 25 beds; obstetric unit, 15 beds; and intensive care unit, 10 beds. Once the assumption of bed interchangeability is dropped, we can no longer lump together the beds of distinct units, as we did in table 5–2. Rather, we should treat each unit as an independent entity—a minihospital, if you will—for the purpose of determining the required excess capacity (or occupancy rate) to ensure a certain protection level. Table 5–4 presents the revised figures for the hypothetical 100-bed hospital.

As can be seen from table 5–4, our hypothetical hospital must maintain an excess capacity of 30 beds (or an occupancy rate of 70 percent) in order to meet the 95 percent protection criterion. Contrast these figures with the corresponding figures given in table 5–2 for a 100-bed hospital: an excess capacity of 16 beds (or an occupancy rate of 84 percent). It is apparent that when hospitals maintain distinct units—and they almost always do—their ability to maintain high occupancy rates is reduced appreciably.

To demonstrate the theoretical basis for the preceding argument, assume that the distinct units of table 5–4 are interchangeable in the sense that a new arrival can be housed in any vacant bed regardless of which unit it happens to be. If we assume that the arrivals of patients in each of the four distinct units

Table 5-4
Revised Excess Capacity Requirement to Ensure a Protection Level of 95 Percent (or Turnaway Rate of 1 day in 20)

Unit	Bed Size	Average Daily Census	Required Excess Capacity		Corresponding Occupancy Rate
			In Beds	In Percentage	
Medical-Surgical	50	39	11	22	78%
Pediatric	25	17	8	32	68
Psychiatric	15	9	6	40	60
Intensive Care	10	5	5	50	50
Total	100	70	30	30	70

is governed by the Poisson process, then the sum of these arrivals itself is a Poisson process. Therefore, the overall bed capacity that satisfies a certain protection level, say, 95 percent, can be determined as follows:

$$P_{(\chi \leqslant k)} = \sum_{\chi=0}^{k} (m^\chi \cdot e^{-m})/\chi! = 0.95$$

Where $P_{(\chi \leqslant k)}$ is the probability that the patient arrivals, on any given day, do not exceed k, and m is the overall average daily census. For the overall average daily census of 70 given in table 5-4, we get:

$$P_{(\chi \leqslant 85)} = \sum_{\chi=0}^{85} (70^\chi \cdot e^{-70})/\chi! = 0.95$$

That is, if 85 beds are set up in response to an overall average daily census of 70, a protection level of 0.95 (95 percent) can be assured, or the chances of overfill limited to 0.05 (5 percent). This implies an occupancy rate of 82 percent, or an excess capacity of 18 percent.

Now assume that the beds set up in distinct units are not interchangeable. The bed capacity now required to ensure that the overfill rate in the medical-surgical unit would be no more than 0.05 (5 percent) is

$$P_{(\chi \leqslant 50)} = \sum_{\chi=0}^{50} (39^\chi \cdot e^{-39})/\chi! = 0.95$$

That is, 50 beds (which implies an occupancy rate of 78 percent) are required to ensure that the overfill rate is not more than 0.05 (5 percent) in the medical-surgical unit. Similarly, it can be shown that the bed requirements of the pediatric, psychiatric, and intensive care units are 25, 15, and 10, respectively. One may pose the question: Why does the total bed requirement of the hospital increase when the assumption of bed interchangeability is lifted? An answer may be found in the law of joint probability. Assume, for the moment, that the patients in the medical-surgical and pediatric units can be switched around, then the probability that *both* units will be full simultaneously is only $0.05^2 = 0.025$. If we further assume that the beds set up in all four units are interchangeable, then the probability that, on any given day, *all* units will be full is infinitesimal: 6.25×10^{-6}. This is another way of saying that if the beds in these units are interchangeable, it is no longer necessary to maintain 100 beds in response to an average daily census of 70, as shown in table 5-4. In fact, we can reduce the bed requirements to 85, and thereby reduce excess capacity to 18 percent (or increase occupancy rate to 82 percent) and still ensure a protection level of 95 percent.

The distribution of beds into the four units in table 5-4 is, of course, arbitrary and may not accord with the real situation. Nonetheless, it is interesting to note that the 1976 occupancy rate of hospitals in size class 100-199 averaged 70.5 percent (see table 5-3).

The Discriminatory Impact of P.L. 93-641

For most industries in the national economy, maximization of capacity utilization is a socially desirable goal shared by all segments of society. Consider, for example, the consequences of raising capacity utilization in the steel industry. The resulting increase in steel production and decrease in unit costs would benefit management in terms of increased profits, labor in terms of higher wages and additional employment, consumers in terms of the lower prices they have to pay for goods that utilize steel, and government in terms of additional tax revenue and a better balance of payment position, and so on. These consequences follow directly from traditional economic theory. Unfortunately, they are so deeply ingrained in the minds of economists that when discussions turn to capacity utilization in the hospital industry, they tend to react as though they are dealing with the steel industry or similar industries.

The beneficial consequences just traced cannot—and should not—be generalized uncritically to the hospital industry. In fact, we have attempted to demonstrate in the earlier sections of this book that optimum capacity utilization in the hospital industry hinges upon the protection level the community seeks, which, in turn, depends on the size of hospitals and the number of distinct units they maintain. If there is substance to the prevailing notion that unutilized capacity is excessive in the hospital industry, establishing a single standard (80 percent occupancy rate) for all hospitals and all localities is certainly not a rational approach to the solution of the problem. In fact, the locational characteristics of the hospital industry point to the conclusion that enforcement of the planning guidelines in their present form would lead to serious regional inequities. In particular, these guidelines seem to discriminate, rather harshly, against rural areas.

There is a preponderance of small hospitals in rural areas and in sparsely populated states such as Texas, Wyoming, Montana, North Dakota, South Dakota, Oklahoma, Idaho, and New Mexico. According to the 1976 hospital census, there are 1,129 hospitals (or 38 percent) with under 50 beds, and 2,240 hospitals (or 69 percent) with under 100 beds in rural areas. The corresponding figures for urban areas are 463 hospitals (or 12 percent) and 1,190 hospitals (or 29 percent), respectively.[13] Thus the typical hospital operating in rural areas has a small bed capacity to begin with and an even smaller bed capacity for the distinct units it may have set up. Going back to tables 5-2 and 5-4, we are struck by the realization that rural hospitals have to reduce their protection levels drastically in order to be in compliance with the occupancy requirement of 80 percent. In addition, unlike urban areas, where alternative facilities are generally available in close proximity, greater distances separate hospitals in rural areas.

Seasonality of Capacity Measures

Beds

Statistical beds (figure 5-14) show the least seasonal fluctuations of any indicator considered in this book ($MA = 0.002$).[14] This is understandable because the number of beds set up and staffed cannot be easily varied in response to temporary ups and downs in demand. Also, as we have seen in the preceding section, hospitals traditionally set up their bed capacity at a certain protection level, that is, a level that accommodates temporay upsurges in demand.

Adult Daily Census

Adult daily census (figure 5-15) is a count of the number of adult and pediatric inpatients on any given day. This indicator reaches its highest levels in January and February and declines fairly steadily until August. There is a mild reversal of the downward trend from August to November. The sharp drop in December is attributable to sociocultural factors such as holidays and vacations. Adult daily census is the best indicator of the level and tempo of inpatient activity experienced by hospitals. Consequently, familiarity with the seasonal pattern

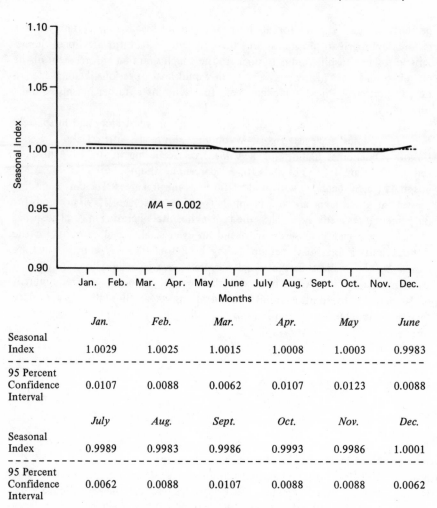

Figure 5-14. Beds

	Jan.	Feb.	Mar.	Apr.	May	June
Seasonal Index	1.0029	1.0025	1.0015	1.0008	1.0003	0.9983
95 Percent Confidence Interval	0.0107	0.0088	0.0062	0.0107	0.0123	0.0088

	July	Aug.	Sept.	Oct.	Nov.	Dec.
Seasonal Index	0.9989	0.9983	0.9986	0.9993	0.9986	1.0001
95 Percent Confidence Interval	0.0062	0.0088	0.0107	0.0088	0.0088	0.0062

of this indicator, including its high and low points, would be helpful to hospital management in improving the effectiveness of their institutions as providers of care and in minimizing wasteful employment of resources.

Adult Occupancy Rate

Adult occupancy rate, or occupancy rate for short, is defined as adult daily census divided by beds, and its complement (1 - occupancy rate) is defined as excess capacity. As we have seen earlier, these two statistics have attracted a great deal of attention in recent times because of their impact on cost. Since

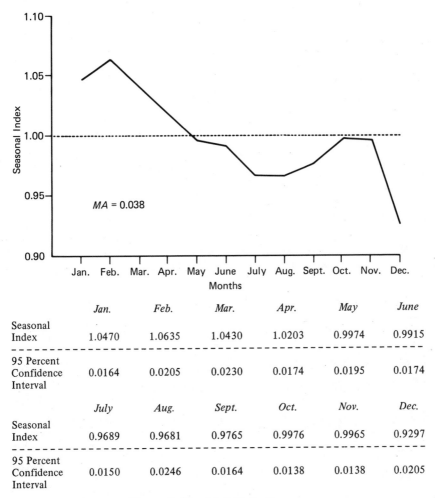

	Jan.	Feb.	Mar.	Apr.	May	June
Seasonal Index	1.0470	1.0635	1.0430	1.0203	0.9974	0.9915
95 Percent Confidence Interval	0.0164	0.0205	0.0230	0.0174	0.0195	0.0174

	July	Aug.	Sept.	Oct.	Nov.	Dec.
Seasonal Index	0.9689	0.9681	0.9765	0.9976	0.9965	0.9297
95 Percent Confidence Interval	0.0150	0.0246	0.0164	0.0138	0.0138	0.0205

Figure 5-15. Adult Daily Census

seasonal fluctuations of beds are minimal (see figure 5-14) Adult occupancy (figure 5-16) traces a pattern which is virtually the "mirror image" of adult daily census. If the hospital management designs the physical layout of the institutions in such a way that it permits some latitude to convert underutilized units for services for which there are temporary upsurges of demand, or to activate and deactivate beds in response to fluctuations in demand, they will have taken a big step toward reducing extreme swings in occupancy rates. Some experiments along these lines have been reported in professional journals. *Hospital Topics* reports a system introduced in a hospital whereby excess maternity beds are utilized for medical overflow by the use of corridor doors which may be

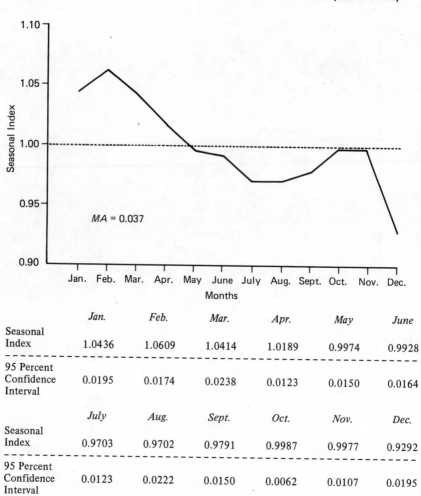

	Jan.	Feb.	Mar.	Apr.	May	June
Seasonal Index	1.0436	1.0609	1.0414	1.0189	0.9974	0.9928
95 Percent Confidence Interval	0.0195	0.0174	0.0238	0.0123	0.0150	0.0164

	July	Aug.	Sept.	Oct.	Nov.	Dec.
Seasonal Index	0.9703	0.9702	0.9791	0.9987	0.9977	0.9292
95 Percent Confidence Interval	0.0123	0.0222	0.0150	0.0062	0.0107	0.0195

Figure 5-16. Adult Occupancy Rate

opened and closed according to need.[15] Some authors have also advocated the use of combined surgery and OB units.[16] An interesting approach proposed recently to deal with the problem of excess capacity in the slack season is the "5-day medical-surgical unit." In such a unit, operations are performed during the week, but cease on weekends. Empty beds are isolated into one unit, and the unit is closed to eliminate staffing requirements for that unit during that 2-day closing period.[17]

Although *active beds* are defined as the overall measure of capacity in the discussions so far, a more adequate definition of *capacity* is the total resources deployed—labor and nonlabor. Some techniques for fuller utilization of capacity

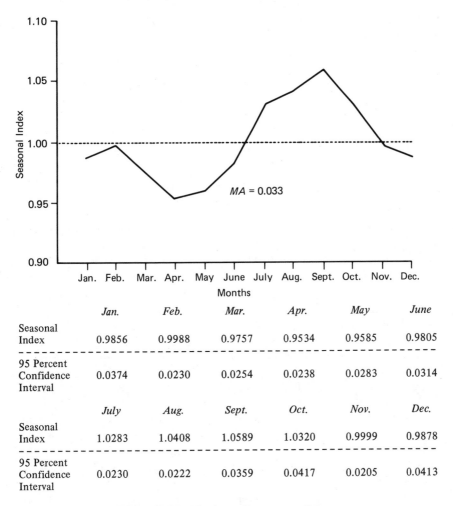

Figure 5-17. Newborn Occupancy Rate

	Jan.	*Feb.*	*Mar.*	*Apr.*	*May*	*June*
Seasonal Index	0.9856	0.9988	0.9757	0.9534	0.9585	0.9805
95 Percent Confidence Interval	0.0374	0.0230	0.0254	0.0238	0.0283	0.0314

	July	*Aug.*	*Sept.*	*Oct.*	*Nov.*	*Dec.*
Seasonal Index	1.0283	1.0408	1.0589	1.0320	0.9999	0.9878
95 Percent Confidence Interval	0.0230	0.0222	0.0359	0.0417	0.0205	0.0413

in its broader sense include (1) employment of part-time nursing personnel at peak periods, (2) closing down nursing stations during slack periods, (3) using floating nurses to cover peak periods, and (4) scheduling elective admissions in such a way as to even out patient loads.

Newborn Occupancy Rate

Since births has a pattern of its own (see figure 5-8), the seasonality of newborn occupancy rate has little in common with that of adult occupancy rate. Indeed, the graph of newborn occupancy rate (figure 5-17) resembles a sine function, with its upswings coinciding roughly with the downswings of adult occupancy rate, and vice versa. Thus, newborn activity operates as a stabilizing force: it moderates extreme fluctuations in the level and tempo of hospital activity. Indeed, the seasonality of newborn, surgical, and outpatient activities, when considered in conjunction with the seasonality of inpatient activity, suggests that, other things being equal, a hospital with a diversified product line can achieve a higher overall occupancy rate than one with a narrow product line. This type of product diversification is somewhat analogous to a firm combining refrigerator and air-conditioner lines with furnaces and stoves.

Surgical Operations

Surgical operations is often used as a crude proxy for product complexity/case severity. A hospitalization episode that entails surgery generally increases per diem expenses as well as length of stay.[18] We have already discussed the relationship between length of stay and expenses per day (figure 5-6). Since each hospitalization episode is associated with a certain level of product complexity/ case severity and a specific length of stay, it is *a propose* to examine the combined effect of these factors on expenses per day.

Figure 5-18 presents a three-dimensional perspective on the combined effect of length of stay and product complexity on expenses per day. Length of stay (LOS) is measured along the horizontal axis, product complexity (PC) is measured along the axis drawn downward and to the left, and expenses per day (EPD) is measured along the vertical axis.

Notice that expenses per day are at a minimum when the hospitalization episode is characterized by the lowest level of product complexity and the lengthiest duration of stay (EPD-1). As the duration of stay shortens and product complexity increases, expenses per day continue to rise, as indicated by EPD-2 and EPD-3. Thus one might say that expenses per day will be at a maximum when the hospitalization episode is characterized by the shortest duration of stay and the highest level of product complexity.

If we turn to figure 5-25, the combined effect of higher levels of product complexity (insofar as they can be deduced from the surgery rates displayed in figure 5-19) and shorter duration of stay (displayed in figure 5-7) is clearly in evidence in the seasonal indexes of adjusted expenses per inpatient day. Notice that the index values given in figure 5-25 are above average during the months of June through August.

What bearing does the foregoing relationship have on expenses per admission? Since expenses per admission are the product of expenses per day and length of stay, the following statements are logical corollaries: expenses per admission will be at a minimum when product complexity is low and duration of stay short, and expenses per admission will be at a maximum when product

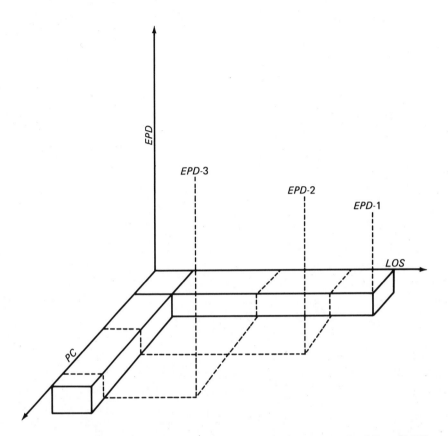

Figure 5-18. The Effects of Product Complexity (*PC*) and Length of Stay (*LOS*) on Expenses per Day (*EPD*)

complexity is high and duration of stay long. Of these, duration of stay exerts greater influence simply because changes in length of stay are measurable only in terms of large, discrete time units—24 hours. The dominant influence of the length of stay factor is clearly in evidence in figure 5-26. Notice that adjusted expenses per admission are below average during the months of June through August, although, as we have seen, per diem expenses are above average during these months.

Seasonality of Surgical Operations

There are several noteworthy features associated with the seasonal pattern of surgical operations (figure 5-19). In the first place, this indicator exhibits the

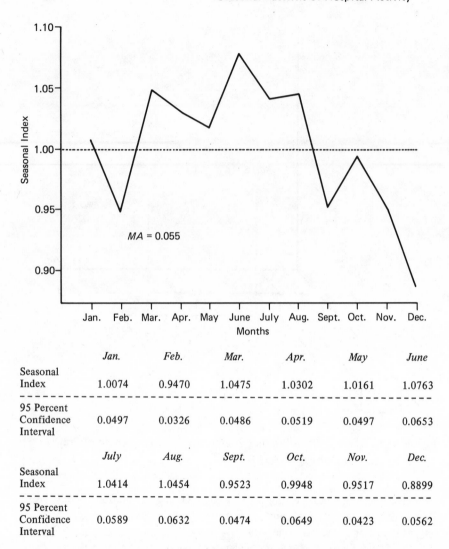

	Jan.	*Feb.*	*Mar.*	*Apr.*	*May*	*June*
Seasonal Index	1.0074	0.9470	1.0475	1.0302	1.0161	1.0763
95 Percent Confidence Interval	0.0497	0.0326	0.0486	0.0519	0.0497	0.0653

	July	*Aug.*	*Sept.*	*Oct.*	*Nov.*	*Dec.*
Seasonal Index	1.0414	1.0454	0.9523	0.9948	0.9517	0.8899
95 Percent Confidence Interval	0.0589	0.0632	0.0474	0.0649	0.0423	0.0562

Figure 5-19. Surgical Operations

greatest seasonal fluctuation of any indicator considered in this book. An *MA* of 0.055 expresses the breadth of upswings and downswings which range from a high of 1.0763 in June to a low of 0.8899 in December.

Surgical activities have upswings and downswings during those periods when inpatient activities have downswings and upswings. Thus the presence of surgical activities operates as a stabilizing force, evening out extreme fluctuations in the overall activity of hospitals. December is a notable exception to this relation.

Surgical operations and outpatient visits, although seemingly unrelated, follow similar patterns of seasonal variations (see figure 5-5). There seems to be a coincidental as well as causative factor involved in this similarity. Incidences of accidents and violence-related injuries are high during the spring and summer months, which partially explain the higher use rate of outpatient facilities during this period. It is also during this period that consumers generally take time off to undergo elective surgery. The causal factor seems to be that injuries resulting from accidents and violence generate the need for surgery.

Revenue Measures

Patient services constitute the primary source of hospital revenue, accounting for close to 96 percent of total revenue. Hospitals, however, do receive revenue from sources not directly related to patient care, such as tuition revenue, unrestricted contributions, parking lot revenue, cafeteria sales, and so forth. Not all revenue recorded is realizable. The nonrealizable portion, or deductions, include charity services, contractual adjustments, personnel adjustments, administrative and policy adjustments, and bad debts. Total recorded revenue (or gross revenue) less deductions equals net revenue. The indicators reported in this section are based on net revenue.

Total Revenue

The major components of total revenue are inpatient revenue and outpatient revenue. It is therefore hardly surprising that the seasonal pattern of total revenue displayed in figure 5-20 is almost identical with that of adjusted patient days (figure 5-2). The only discernible difference is in the index value for December, which is slightly higher for total revenue. This may be due, in part at any rate, to year-end accounting adjustments.

Revenue per Adjusted Patient Day

Fluctuations in revenue per adjusted patient day (figure 5-21) are less pronounced than most other indicators with the index values of all months close to 1.0000. The reason for this uniformity is the fact that the major component of revenue per adjusted patient day is routine service charges (room rate), which remain generally fixed during the year. The index values are slightly above average during June through September, and reach their peak in December.

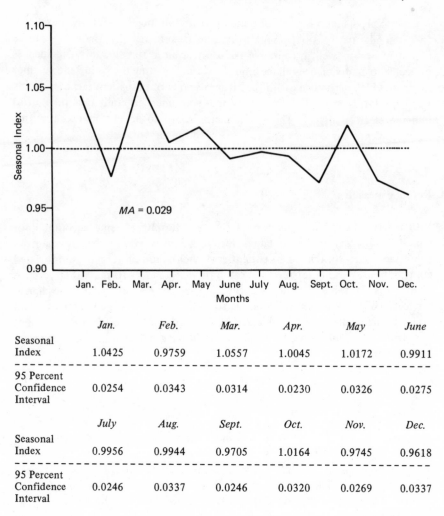

	Jan.	Feb.	Mar.	Apr.	May	June
Seasonal Index	1.0425	0.9759	1.0557	1.0045	1.0172	0.9911
95 Percent Confidence Interval	0.0254	0.0343	0.0314	0.0230	0.0326	0.0275

	July	Aug.	Sept.	Oct.	Nov.	Dec.
Seasonal Index	0.9956	0.9944	0.9705	1.0164	0.9745	0.9618
95 Percent Confidence Interval	0.0246	0.0337	0.0246	0.0320	0.0269	0.0337

Figure 5-20. Total Revenue

Revenue per Adjusted Admission

Unlike revenue per adjusted patient day, which exhibits minimal seasonal fluctuations, revenue per adjusted admission (figure 5-22) displays a seasonal pattern quite similar to that of adult length of stay—high in winter and low in summer. Indeed, if one ignores the slight divergence that occurs in the month of December, the similarity between the two graphs is almost perfect. (see figure 5-7). Figure 5-6 furnishes the explanation for this similarity. Notice that *EPA*

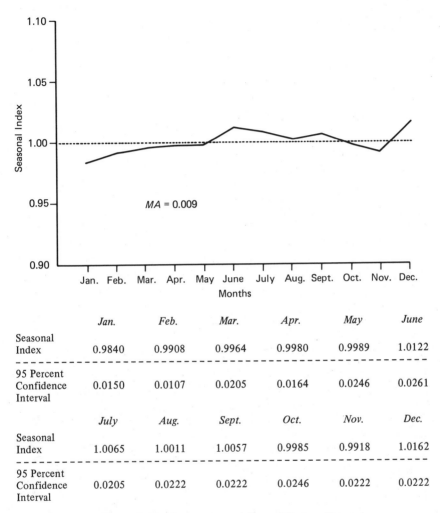

	Jan.	Feb.	Mar.	Apr.	May	June
Seasonal Index	0.9840	0.9908	0.9964	0.9980	0.9989	1.0122
95 Percent Confidence Interval	0.0150	0.0107	0.0205	0.0164	0.0246	0.0261
	July	Aug.	Sept.	Oct.	Nov.	Dec.
Seasonal Index	1.0065	1.0011	1.0057	0.9985	0.9918	1.0162
95 Percent Confidence Interval	0.0205	0.0222	0.0222	0.0246	0.0222	0.0222

Figure 5-21. Revenue per Adjusted Patient Day

(expenses per admission) varies directly with length of stay. Consequently, the revenue charged per admission also varies directly with length of stay.

Expense Measures

The expense statistics reported by the American Hospital Association, its constituents, and allied health associations are total expenses, adjusted expenses per

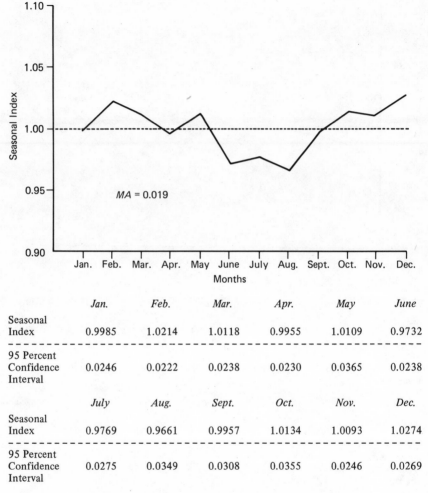

	Jan.	Feb.	Mar.	Apr.	May	June
Seasonal Index	0.9985	1.0214	1.0118	0.9955	1.0109	0.9732
95 Percent Confidence Interval	0.0246	0.0222	0.0238	0.0230	0.0365	0.0238
	July	Aug.	Sept.	Oct.	Nov.	Dec.
Seasonal Index	0.9769	0.9661	0.9957	1.0134	1.0093	1.0274
95 Percent Confidence Interval	0.0275	0.0349	0.0308	0.0355	0.0246	0.0269

Figure 5-22. Revenue per Adjusted Admission

inpatient day, and adjusted expenses per admission. As discussed in chapter 2, the last two statistics are estimates of expenses per day and expenses per admission, respectively. Over the years, these measures have achieved a high level of visibility, recognition, and acceptance.

Components of Total Expenses

Like the total expenses incurred by all industries, total expenses incurred by the hospital industry are the product of two factors: (1) the expenses of producing

Table 5-5
Effect of Unit Expenses and Quantity Produced on Total Expenses:
Community Hospitals

1	2	3	4	5
Year	Expenses per Unit of Output (Adjusted Patient Day)	Total Quantity of Output Produced (Total Adjusted Patient Days)	Total Expenses (Col. 2 × Col. 3)	Increase
1970	$ 73.73	265.3 million	$19.56 billion	—
1976	$151.28	298.2 million	$45.11 billion	$25.55 billion

Source: American Hospital Association, *Hospital Statistics,* 1977 ed., Table 1. Reprinted with permission.

a unit of output, and (2) the quantity of output produced. For illustrative purposes, let us assume, for the moment, that adjusted patient day is an appropriate unit of output. We can now show the combined effect of expenses per unit of output and the quantity of output produced (table 5-5).

From table 5-5 we see that total expenses incurred by the hospital industry is the product of unit expenses and the quantity of output produced. From 1970 to 1976, total expenses increased by $25.55 billion. According to the values shown in table 5-5, roughly 89.5 percent of this increase is due to expense increase and 10.5 percent is due to quantity increase.[19] To anticipate the discussions that follow, this disaggregation underestimates the effect of quantity increase because of the inappropriateness of adjusted patient day as a uniform (homogeneous) measure of hospital output.

Adjusted Patient Day as an Output Measure

The unit of measure of an adjusted patient day is a 24-hour timespan without regard to what goes on during that timespan. If the "contents" of that timespan, that is, the number and quantities of services provided per day, change, as indeed they do, an adjusted patient day pertaining to one time period is not comparable to an adjusted patient day pertaining to another time period. Therefore, adjusted patient day is not an appropriate output unit for the measurement of pure expense changes of hospital services. When we deal with tangible products, the logic of this argument becomes so compelling, so self-evident, as to need no elaboration. We do not, for example, measure price changes of milk by pricing 1 gallon of milk in 1977 and $1\frac{1}{2}$ gallons of milk in 1978 and noting the difference. Yet it is precisely this type of comparison that one makes when changes in adjusted expenses per inpatient day are interpreted as changes in expenses per unit of output in the hospital industry.

The Essential Nature of Adjusted Expenses
per Inpatient Day/Admission

One often encounters graphs such as the one in figure 5-23 accompanied by tables and interpretative statements designed to drive home the notion that expenses (prices) of hospital services are rising much faster than other goods and services. Here, for example, is an excerpt from a recent publication:

> In 1965, the average expense per stay was $311; by 1974, this had almost tripled to $873. . . . This increase is all the more remarkable since the average length of hospital stay declined steadily from 1969 through 1974; thus, the average expense per day in the hospital has actually risen more rapidly.[20]

The juxtaposition of consumer price index (CPI) and adjusted expenses per inpatient day is a palpably misleading procedure. This is not simply because the former measures "price" changes while the latter measures "expense" changes. The difference is more fundamental. The CPI measures the price changes of a *fixed* quantity of goods and services, while adjusted expenses per inpatient day measures the expense changes of a steadily *increasing* quantity of services. For example, from 1969 to 1976 the following increases in the quantities of services provided per typical adjusted patient day have been observed:

Nuclear medicine procedures:	373%
Occupational therapy manhours:	171
Pharmaecutical items utilized:	149
Intravenous therapy manhours:	133
Inhalation therapy manhours:	124
Clinical laboratory tests:	113
Physical therapy treatments:	81
Therapeutic radiology procedures:	60
Diagnostic radiology procedures:	54

Thus adjusted expenses per inpatient day includes the combined effects of expense increases and quantity increases, and so does adjusted expenses per admission. An unfortunate aspect of using adjusted expenses per inpatient day/admission as a measure of inflation in the hospital sector is the fact that it shifts the focus of attention away from the more potent cause of hospital expenditure increase—escalating demand—and toward what is probably a somewhat less important and certainly a less controllable cause—inflation. It is as though

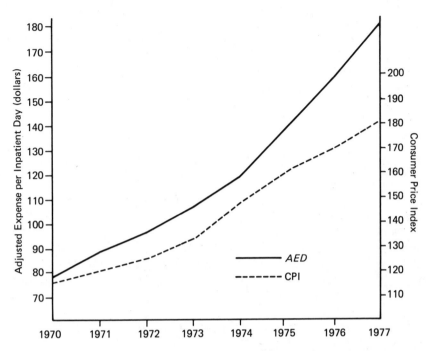

Sources: American Hospital Association, *Hospital Statistics,* 1977 ed. and 1978 ed. (reprinted by permission); and U.S. Dept. of Commerce, Bureau of Labor Statistics.

Figure 5-23. Annual Trend: Adjusted Expenses per Inpatient Day (*AED*) and
        Consumer Price Index (*CPI*)

the problem of rising hospital expenditures would disappear if only the hospital industry could be persuaded to become more efficient in a technical sense, that is, convert inputs into hospital outputs at minimum cost.

The Hospital Cost Index (HCI) and the
Hospital Intensity Index (HII)

In an attempt to provide a better persepctive on hospital services and expenses, the American Hospital Association introduced, in 1976, two new statistics—hospital cost index (HCI) and hospital intensity index (HII). Both these indexes were originally based of thirty-seven specific services or components which have been enlarged to forty-six in 1978. The HCI tracks the cost changes of a *fixed quantity* of these components; and the HII tracks the *quantity changes* of these components.[21]

From 1970 to 1977, HCI rose at an average annual rate of 7.9 percent as opposed to a rate of increase of 12.8 registered by adjusted expenses per inpatient day. The rate of increase of HII averaged 4.2 percent. It is the position of the AHA that if one wishes to compare the rate of inflation in the hospital sector vis-à-vis the rest of the economy, it is the movement of HCI (and not adjusted expenses per inpatient day) that should be compared with the CPI or any other index of general inflation.

Adjusted Patient Days Weighted by Service Intensity

For an accurate measurement of changes in the quantity of service provided by the hospital industry, it is necessary to weight adjusted patient days by the intensity factor. Table 5-6 presents adjusted patient days in 1970 and 1976 weighted by HII.

Notice that while adjusted patient days increased by 32.9 million (or 12.4 percent), adjusted patient days weighted by HII increased by 125.1 million (or 43.0 percent). If we disaggregate the components of total expenses by substituting the values given in column 4 for quantity and working out the results as shown in, note 19, we obtain the following results:[22]

Expense effect: $15.01 billion, or 58.7 percent

Quantity effect: $10.54 billion, or 41.3 percent

Factors Contributing Toward Rising Hospital Expenses

We are now in a position to see the phenomenon of escalating hospital expenses in perspective. To recapitulate the findings of the preceding section, the contributary factors are:

1. *Inflation.* Inflation increases the costs of labor and nonlabor resources

Table 5-6
Real Effect of Unit Expenses and Quantity Produced on Total Expenses:
Community Hospitals

1	2	3	4	5	6	7
Year	Total Adjusted Patient Days	HII	Total Quantity of Output Produced (Col. 2 × Col. 3)	Total Expenses	Expenses per Unit of Output (Col. 3 – Col. 4)	Increase in Total Expenses
1970	265.3 million	1.0961	290.8 million	$19.56 billion	$ 67.26	—
1976	298.2 million	1.3948	415.9 million	$45.11 billion	$108.46	$25.55 billion

Source: American Hospital Association, *Hospital Statistics, 197   d.* Reprinted with permission.

purchased by hospitals for the production of hospital care. As noted earlier, annual inflation rate in the hospital sector averages 7.9 percent.[23]

2. *Quantity Increase.* Quantity increase is the resultant of two factors: (a) *intensity increase,* that is, increase in the quantity of services provided per typical patient day (as noted earlier, intensity has been rising at an average annual rate of 4.2 percent); and (b) *volume increase.* Returning to table 5-6, we note that during 1970-76, adjusted patient days rose from 265.3 million to 298.2 million, or an increase of 32.9 million. This increase may be attributed to demographic trends[24] and higher per capita utilization of hospital care by the population.[25]

When we consider these factors, it becomes readily apparent that, contrary to popular belief, it is not inflation alone, but the combined effect of inflation and the burgeoning consumption of hospital care, that exacerbates the rate of increase in national hospital expenditures.

Seasonality of Expense Measures

Total Expenses

One would have expected fluctuations in total expenses (figure 5-24) to be in line with fluctuations in the volume of services—adjusted patient days. This is true only up to a point (see figure 5-2). An MA of 0.018 indicates that variations in total expenses are less pronounced than those of adjusted patient days. Why is this so? As pointed out earlier (chapter 1), fixed costs constitute a substantial portion of total costs of hospitals.[26] Since fixed costs, by definition, do not vary from month to month, the presence of a large fixed-cost component moderates fluctuations in total expenses. However, in a general sense, the seasonal pattern of total expenses conforms to the seasonal pattern of adjusted patient days, except for the month of December, when the expense index diverges from the volume index presumably due to year-end accounting adjustments.

Adjusted Expenses per Inpatient Day

If we superimpose on figure 5-25, the graph pertaining to adult occupancy rate (figure 5-16) turned upside down, the two graphs almost coincide. This is indicative of the strong negative relationship between expenses per unit of output and occupancy rate in the hospital industry. The higher the occupancy rate, the lower the expenses per unit of output and conversely. One could also observe a negative relationship between expenses per adjusted patient day and adult

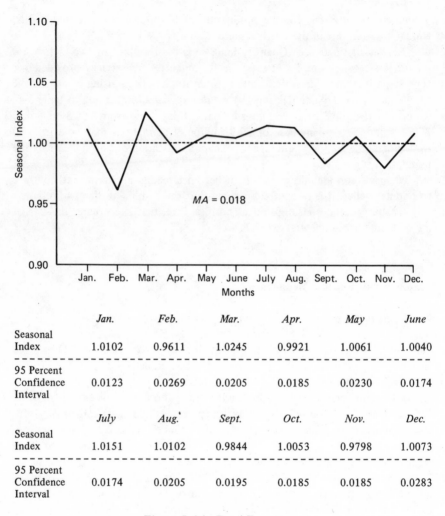

	Jan.	Feb.	Mar.	Apr.	May	June
Seasonal Index	1.0102	0.9611	1.0245	0.9921	1.0061	1.0040
95 Percent Confidence Interval	0.0123	0.0269	0.0205	0.0185	0.0230	0.0174

	July	Aug.	Sept.	Oct.	Nov.	Dec.
Seasonal Index	1.0151	1.0102	0.9844	1.0053	0.9798	1.0073
95 Percent Confidence Interval	0.0174	0.0205	0.0195	0.0185	0.0185	0.0283

Figure 5-24. Total Expenses

length of stay (figure 5-7). The shorter the length of stay, the higher generally are per diem expenses.

Adjusted Expenses per Admission

One would have expected a very close correspondence between the seasonal patterns of adjusted expenses per admission (figure 5-26) and adult length of stay (figure 5-7). Although these patterns have basic similarities, they are not all

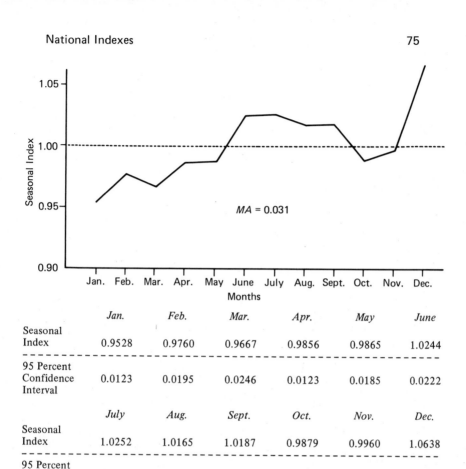

	Jan.	Feb.	Mar.	Apr.	May	June
Seasonal Index	0.9528	0.9760	0.9667	0.9856	0.9865	1.0244
95 Percent Confidence Interval	0.0123	0.0195	0.0246	0.0123	0.0185	0.0222
	July	Aug.	Sept.	Oct.	Nov.	Dec.
Seasonal Index	1.0252	1.0165	1.0187	0.9879	0.9960	1.0638
95 Percent Confidence Interval	0.0230	0.0195	0.0185	0.0174	0.0205	0.0302

Figure 5-25. Adjusted Expenses per Inpatient Day

that striking. For example, the substantial drop in length of stay in June, July, and August is not matched by a corresponding decline in per admission expenses. There are two reasons why the expense indexes do not decline as much as the length of stay indexes. First, turning to figure 5-16, we notice that occupancy rate is unusually low during the months of June, July, and August, and, as we have seen, lower occupancy rates tend to increase expenses per unit of output. Second, these months are also characterized by high levels of surgical operations (figure 5-19), indicators of case severity/complexity. It would therefore seem that the reduction in adjusted expenses per inpatient admission which shorter stays would have normally brought about is partially offset by excess capacity and case severity/complexity.

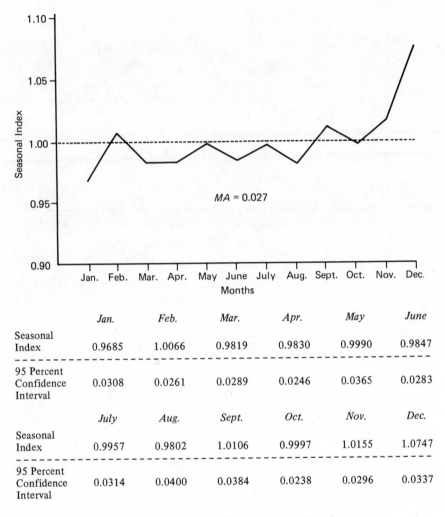

	Jan.	Feb.	Mar.	Apr.	May	June
Seasonal Index	0.9685	1.0066	0.9819	0.9830	0.9990	0.9847
95 Percent Confidence Interval	0.0308	0.0261	0.0289	0.0246	0.0365	0.0283
	July	Aug.	Sept.	Oct.	Nov.	Dec.
Seasonal Index	0.9957	0.9802	1.0106	0.9997	1.0155	1.0747
95 Percent Confidence Interval	0.0314	0.0400	0.0384	0.0238	0.0296	0.0337

Figure 5-26. Adjusted Expenses per Admission

Notes

1. These values are reported in "Hospital Indicators," *Hospitals,* May 16, 1977. Reprinted with permission.

2. This is a very rough measure of stability because the assumption that the index has been computed from a distribution arising out of a random process does not hold.

3. See note 7 in chapter 1.

4. U.S. Department of Health, Education and Welfare, Public Health Service, *Health United States 1976-77,* DHEW Pub. No. (HRA)77-1232, p. 215.

5. P. Pasamanick, S. Danitz, and H. Knoblock, "Socio-economic and Seasonal Variations in Birth Rates," *Milbank Mem. Fund Quart.* 38 (July 1960).

6. K. Chang, S. Chan, W. Low, and C. Ng, "Climate and Conception Rates in Hong Kong," *Human Biol.* 35 (Sept. 1963).

7. Note that turnover rate of babies (TOR_b) may be defined as a function of newborn occupancy rate (OR_n) and newborn length of stay (LOS_n). That is,

$$TOR_b = \frac{\text{newborn admissions}}{\text{bassinets}} = \frac{OR_n \times 365}{LOS_n}$$

8. V.P. Barbba, "Population Trends and the Cost of Medical Care," *U.S. Dept. of Commerce News,* Washington, July 29, 1976.

9. National Academy of Sciences, Institute of Medicine, *Controlling the Supply of Hospital Beds: A Policy Statement,* Washington, 1976.

10. See "National Guidelines for Health Planning," *Federal Register* 43 (March 28, 1978):13040-50.

11. The "Planning Guidelines" provide for certain exceptions, but they are both vague and perfunctory.

12. If we assume that patient arrivals are Poisson distributed, the probability that x number of patients will arrive on any given day is

$$P_{(x)} = (m^x \cdot e^{-m})/x!$$

where m is the mean number of arrivals per day. The probability that the number of arrivals on any given day will be less than or equal to a certain number, say, k, is:

$$P_{(x \leqslant k)} = \sum_{x=0}^{k} (m^x \cdot e^{-m})/x!$$

and the probability that the number of patient arrivals on any given day will exceed k is

$$P_{(x > k)} = 1 - P_{(x \leqslant k)}$$

13. American Hospital Association, *Comparative Statistics of Health Facilities and Population: Metropolitan and Nonmetropolitan Areas,* 1978 ed., p. 20.

We have assumed that "urban" and "rural" are roughly coterminous with SMSA and nonSMSA. Reprinted with permission.

14. See the last section of chapter 2 for a definition of statistical beds.

15. M.S. Beaulieu, "Dual-Purpose OB Unit: Alice Peck Day Memorial Hospital, Lebanon, New Hampshire," *Hospital Topics* (May 1966): 118-19.

16. F. Gordon, "Why Not Join Surgery with the Obstetrical Unit?" *Modern Hospital* (Aug. 1967):115-18.

17. "Feasibility of a 5-Day Medical-Surgical Unit, *Hospital Administration Currents* 21 (Jan.-Feb. 1977):1-4.

18. See Commission on Professional and Hospital Activities, *Length of Stay in PAS Hospitals, by Diagnosis, United States, 1975,* Ann Arbor, Oct. 1977.

19. Let E and ΔE denote 1970 expenses per adjusted patient day and 1970-1976 increase in expenses per adjusted patient day, respectively. Let Q and ΔQ denote 1970 adjusted patient days and 1970-1976 increase in adjusted patient days, respectively. Then the 1970-1976 increase in total expenses (ΔTE) can be disaggregated as follows (m = million):

ΔTE = Expense effect + quantity effect + interaction effect

$\quad = \Delta EQ + \Delta QE + \Delta E\Delta Q$

$\quad = (\$77.55 \times 265.3 \text{ m}) + (32.9 \text{ m} \times \$73.73) + (\$77.55 \times \$32.9 \text{ m})$

$\quad = \$20{,}574.0 \text{ m} + \$2{,}425.7 \text{ m} + \$2{,}551.4 \text{ m}$

If we apportion the interaction effect between expense effect and quantity effect on a pro rata basis, we have

Expense effect = (20,574.0 m + \$2,283.5 m) = \$22,857.5 m   (89.5%)

Quantity effect = (\$2,425.7 m + \$267.9 m)   = \$ 2,693.6 m   (10.5%)

Total = \$25,551.1 m (100.0%)

20. Council on Wage and Price Stability, *The Complex Puzzle of Rising Health Care Costs: Can the Private Sector Fit it Together?* (prepared by Paul S. McAuliffe, Deputy General Counsel, with the research assistance of Susanne J. Tierney), Washington, DC, Dec. 1976, p. 73.

21. For detailed information on the HCI and the HII, see the following references: P.J. Phillip et al., *The Nature of Hospital Costs: Three Studies,* Hospital Research and Educational Trust, Chicago, 1976; P.J. Phillip. "HCI/HII— Two New AHA Indexes Measure Costs, Intensity," *Hosp. Fin. Mgt.* (April 1977): 20-26; P.J. Phillip, "New AHA Indexes Provide Fairer View of Rising Costs," *Hospitals* (July 16, 1977):175-82.

22. For a comparable breakdown, see M. Feldstein and A. Taylor, *The*

Rapid Rise of Hospital Costs, Council on Wage and Price Stability, Staff Report, January 1977, pp. 24-28.

23. Strictly speaking, the rate of increase in HCI can be equated with inflation only in the limiting case in which productivity in the hospital industry remains unchanged. If productivity is rising, HCI underestimates inflation rate; and if productivity is falling, HCI overestimates inflation rate. Nonetheless, the movement of HCI provides a better measure of inflation rate in the hospital industry than anything else currently available.

24. The population of the United States is growing at an annual rate of about 0.8 percent; and the number of people 65 years and over is increasing at an annual rate of about 2.4 percent.

25. Rising standard of living, more pervasive health insurance coverage, better access to care thanks to social programs such as Medicare and Medicaid, and the causal relation between technological innovations and demand all contribute to rising consumption of hospital services.

26. Empirical studies on hospital costs have produced estimates of fixed cost ranging from 50 to 80 percent of total cost. An explanation offered for this wide variation in the results obtained has to do with the *time period* used by researchers. The shorter the time period used, the higher will be the estimate of fixed cost, and vice versa. For in the very long run, all costs are variable. (See J.R. Lave and L.B. Lave, "Estimated Cost Functions for Pennsylvania Hospitals," *Inquiry* VII (June 1970):3-32.

6

Treatment of Regional Differences

Regional Variations

The discussions so far have been in terms of national indexes, that is, indexes constructed from national data. How generalizable are these indexes to constituent segments of the hospital universe, such as census regions, states, metropolitan areas, and individual hospitals? It is necessary to explore this aspect of seasonality before one can make definitive statements about the extent to which the seasonal indexes developed in this study can be used by the constituent segments of the hospital universe.

It was pointed out earlier that seasonal variations are caused by climatic and sociocultural factors. While the sociocultural factors may be taken as more or less uniform across the country, the same cannot be said of climatic factors. Continental United States, stretching as it does from roughly $25°$ to $50°$ north latitude and from $65°$ and $125°$ west longitude, covers several temperature and pressure zones. The topographical features of the country include mountains, hills, plateaus, valleys, plains, lowlands, and sea coasts. All these cause regional differences in climatic conditions typified by the Snow Belt, the Sun Belt, the Prairies, the Savannas, the Great American Desert, and so on. The two noncontiguous states—Alaska and Hawaii—accentuate these regional differences. The former stretches into the arctic tundra, while the latter enjoys climatic conditions characteristic of tropical islands.

Because of these reasons, it is unlikely that the national indexes developed in this study will be appropriate to all constituent parts of the hospital universe. It is possible, for example, that the seasonal patterns of certain indicators pertaining to a specific region, state, metropolitan area, or hospital might deviate from national patterns.

Indexes Specific to Census Regions

The U.S. Bureau of Census has established nine census regions, each composed of contiguous states.[1] It is reasonable to expect a degree of uniformity in the climatic conditions of states that constitute a census region.[2] Accordingly, we have constructed seasonal indexes specific to each census region in addition to the national indexes. These are presented in tables 7-1 through 7-10. The measures of amplitude pertaining to these indexes are provided in table 7-11.

Although the need to furnish more accurate seasonal indexes for the users' specific area of interest led to the development of regional indexes, an examination of these indexes and associated measures of amplitude is instructive in itself. For example, regional seasonality, when studied in relation to one another and to the nation as a whole, can provide valuable insights into the effects of climate, demography, topography, style of care, and their interaction on the seasonal pattern of hospital indicators pertaining to regions. Of course, an incisive analysis along these lines would require much greater knowledge of regional characteristics than we have. Therefore, we will confine ourselves to a discussion of the more salient regional differences and the possible reasons that contribute to these differences. It should be emphasized that the reasons advanced are speculative and tentative rather than categorical and definitive. Indeed, users who are more familiar with the characteristics and peculiarities of their regions may find reasons other than the ones we have advanced, and may uncover reasons we overlooked. In any event, the discussions that follow will hopefully stimulate interest in studies focusing on the impact of climatic, demographic, topographic, socioeconomic, and institutional factors on the pattern of hospital utilization.

Overall Variations

If we focus on the columns of table 7-11 that list the measures of amplitude of individual census regions, we notice that the overall variation is least in census region 9 (Pacific). See figure 6-1. If we ignore Alaska, which has very few hospitals and beds, the states that constitute the Pacific region enjoy a relatively mild, equable climate.[3] Since climatic variation is one of the principal determinants of seasonality, the smaller variations that characterize the Pacific region are probably due in part to the relatively equable climate that prevails in this region. Demographic characteristics may also be a contributory factor. The Pacific region has a relatively lower proportion of older people who are more susceptible to climatic variations. According to the Bureau of the Census, the percentages of the population 65 years and over and 75 years and over in census region 9 are 9.1 and 3.5, respectively, compared with 9.9 and 3.8 for the nation as a whole.[4]

The census regions that exhibit the widest month-to-month fluctuations are region 7 (West South Central) and region 5 (East South Central). See figures 6-2 and 6-3, respectively. Notice that the measures of amplitude pertaining to these regions are larger than the national values for virtually all hospital indicators. Also noteworthy is the striking similarity between the graphs pertaining to regions 7 and 5.

It is significant that regions 7 and 5 make up the southernmost part of the United States, with climatic conditions somewhat different from those that

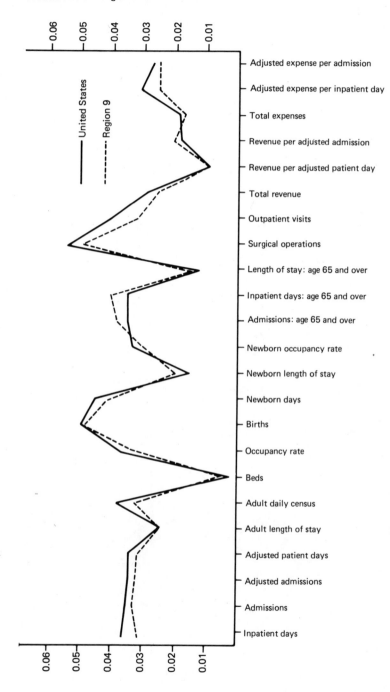

Figure 6-1. Measures of Amplitude: United States and Region 9 (Pacific)

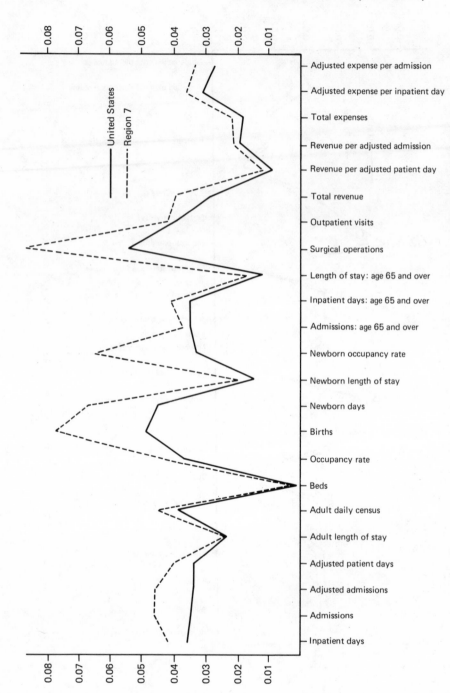

Figure 6–2. Measures of Amplitude: United States and Region 7 (West South Central)

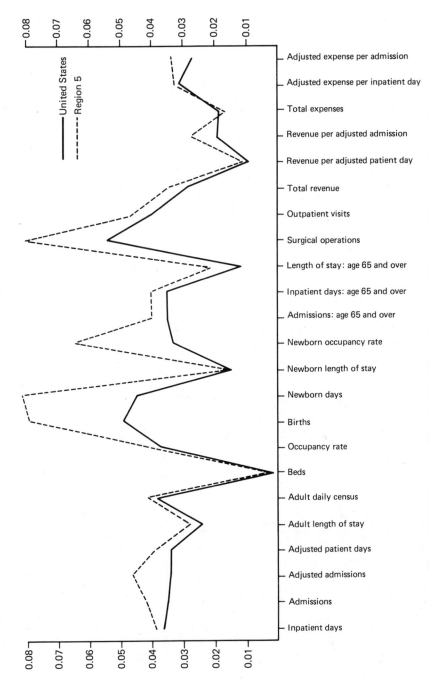

Figure 6–3. Measures of Amplitude: United States and Region 5 (East South Central)

Table 6-1
Selected Characteristics of Census Regions

Characteristic	United States	Census Regions								
		1	2	3	4	5	6	7	8	9
Personal income per capita[a]	$6,441	$6,590	$6,932	$6,007	$6,793	$5,194	$6,130	$5,895	$5,990	$7,071
Percent of households below poverty level[b]	14.7%	11.0%	12.4%	17.1%	12.0%	23.9%	15.3%	21.3%	15.3%	12.1%
Number of nonfederal physicians per 100,000 population[c]	174	222	216	169	151	123	146	134	161	210

[a]U.S. Department of Commerce, Bureau of Economic Analysis, *Survey of Current Business 57*, Washington, April 1977.

[b]U.S. Department of Commerce, *General Social and Economic Characteristics, United States Summary*, PC(1)-C1, U.S. Govt. Printing Office, Washington, June 1972.

[c]L.J. Goodman, *Physician Distribution in the U.S., 1976*, American Medical Association, Center for Health Services Research and Development, Chicago, 1977.

prevail in the northern part of the country. Furthermore, as table 6-1 shows, these regions are characterized by the lowest personnel income per capita, the highest percentage of households below the poverty level, and the lowest number of physicians per capita. It is therefore apparent that the characteristics of a region impact on the level of fluctuations in hospital utilization. The nature of this impact is a subject that merits further investigation. In this connection, an interesting hypothesis that suggests itself is the following: the greater the scarcity of physicians in a region, the higher will be the month-to-month fluctuations in the level of hospital activity. There is an a priori basis to assume that this may be the case. While hospital management would prefer an even level of activity, physicians have a role in the scheudling of patients, particularly the nonemergency and elective cases. When physicians are scarce, their preferences concerning the hospitalization of patients, which may not mesh with those of hospital management, are likely to be more decisive.

Variations of Individual Indicators

If we focus on a specific indicator given in table 7-11 and examine its seasonal pattern across census regions, the following typologies emerge: (1) indicators whose seasonal patterns remain virtually unchanged across regions; (2) indicators whose general "shapes" or "configurations" remain the same, but whose peaks and troughs appear in an exaggerated or attenuated form; and (3) indicators whose "shapes" or "configurations" are not the same in all regions.

Type 1 Indicators

Indicators whose seasonal patterns remain virtually unchanged across regions include adult length of stay, adult occupancy rate, and beds. Figure 6-4 displays the seasonal pattern of adult length of stay for the nation as a whole and for census region 4 (East North Central). Notice the close conformity. A similar degree of conformity is observed for adult occupancy rate and beds. It is significant that if we rank order all the hospital indicators included in this book in terms of the degree of endogenous control, these type 1 indicators would probably be at the top of the list. For example, hospital administrators/staff physicians have far greater control over beds, adult occupancy rate, and adult length of stay than they have over, say, admissions, outpatient visits, surgical operations, and adjusted expenses per inpatient day. Therefore, one may advance the hypothesis that the greater the degree of endogenous control, the greater would be the uniformity of seasonality across regions.

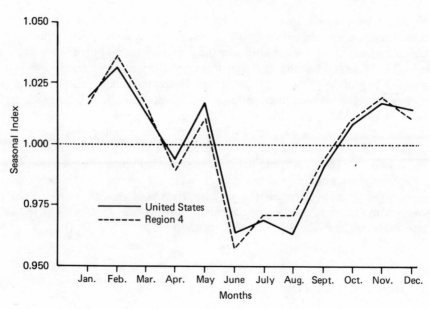

Figure 6-4. Adult Length of Stay: United States and Region 4 (East North Central)

Type 2 Indicators

Type 2 indicators, which comprise the largest group, include inpatient days, admissions, adjusted admissions, adjusted patient days, adult daily census, births, newborn days, newborn length of stay, newborn occupancy rate, total revenue, revenue per adjusted patient day, revenue per adjusted admission, total expenses, adjusted expenses per inpatient day, and adjusted expenses per admission. In what follows we will examine the more important instances, where peaks and troughs of an indicator appear in an exaggerated or attenuated form.

Adult Daily Census. A question that calls for an answer is: Why does adult daily census fall in type 2 in view of the fact that adult occupancy rate, which is placed in type 1, is defined as adult daily census divided by beds? An answer may be found in the concept of statistical beds introduced in chapter 2. Hospitals do have some limited latitude to vary bed capacity in response to temporary ups and downs in demand. The effect of this action is to moderate extreme fluctuations in adult occupancy rate. Table 6-2 presents an illustrative example. Notice that fluctuations in *OR* (occupancy rate) are less pronounced than *OR'*, the fluctuations that would have prevailed had bed capacity been kept constant at 100.

Table 6–2
Effect of Statistical Beds on Occupancy Rate

1	2	3	4	5	6
Period	Average Daily Census	Initial Beds	Statistical Beds	OR' (Col. 2 ÷ Col. 3)	OR (Col. 2 ÷ Col. 4)
Period 1	80	100	100	80%	80%
Period 2	60	100	95	60%	63%
Period 3	95	100	105	95%	90%

Figure 6–5 displays the national indexes for adult daily census overlayed upon those for region 8, the Mountain states. It is apparent that region 8 experiences a higher level of inpatient activity during the winter months. A variety of reasons for this accentuated winter upswing suggest themselves. The relatively low percentage of the population in region 8 residing in metropolitan areas combined with the generally low density of population in the region imply that patients must travel greater distances to seek care. When we consider the rough-

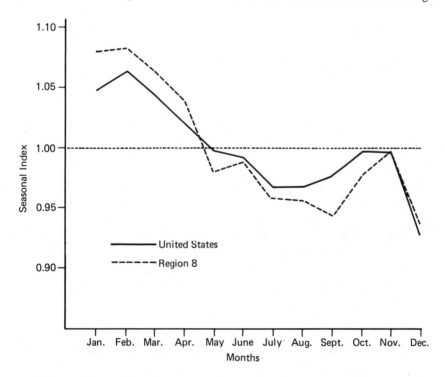

Figure 6–5. Adult Daily Census: United States and Region 8 (Mountain)

ness of the terrain, the severity of the climate, and the very real threat of winter road closures in the higher elevations, it becomes apparent that in many cases outpatient management of noncritical conditions would be difficult. Some evidence in support of this hypothesis is provided by Gornick, who concludes, "Evidently, where distances to health care resources are relatively great, more health care is provided on an inpatient basis than where the distances to services are less."[5]

The preceding line of reasoning is supported by the high adult length of stay experienced in region 8 during January and February. For the 65 and over age group in particular, length of stay is markedly higher in January, February, March, and May. This may well be indicative of a reluctance on the part of physicians to discharge patients early because of the difficulty those patients would have in obtaining followup care on an ambulatory basis.

Births. In figure 6-6 the indexes specific to region 5 (East South Central) are superimposed on the national indexes. Notice that the peak in autumn and the trough in spring appear in an exaggerated form in region 5. In contrast, consider figure 6-7, where the indexes specific to region 1 (New England) are shown

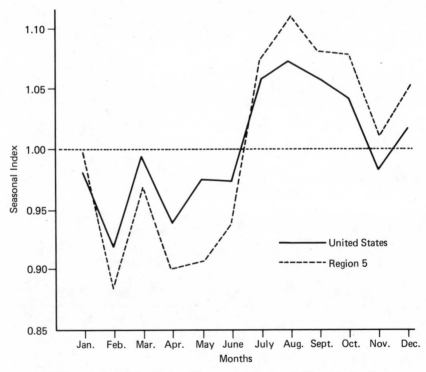

Figure 6-6. Births: United States and Region 5 (New England)

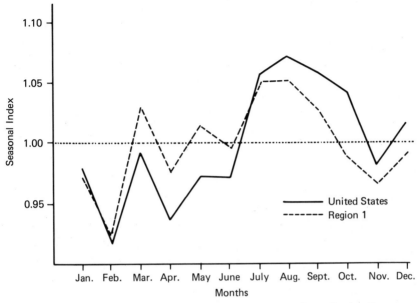

Figure 6-7. Births: United States and Region 1 (New England)

along with the national indexes. The peaks and troughs of New England, a region characterized by milder summers, appear in an attenuated form. Thus figures 6-6 and 6-7 provide striking confirmation of the effect of climatic conditions on conception rates discussed earlier (chapters 1 and 5). Other newborn indicators, such as newborn days and newborn occupancy rate, parallel the fluctuations of births displayed in figures 6-6 and 6-7.

In order to bring out more clearly the influence of climate on newborn utilization pattern, we have combined the census regions that lie in the extreme north of the country into one region and the census regions that lie in the extreme south of the country into another region. Average indexes of births and newborn days are then computed and displayed in table 6-3. Notice that new-

Table 6-3
Influence of Climate on Newborn Utilization Pattern

Indicator	Spring (Mar., Apr., May)		Autumn (Sept., Oct., Nov.)	
	Regions 1, 2, 4	Regions 5, 7	Regions 1, 2, 4	Regions 5, 7
Births	0.9883	0.9210	1.0213	1.0576
Newborn Days	0.9897	0.9259	1.0105	1.0605

born utilization is substantially lower in the spring in the southern region than it is in the northern region. In contrast, newborn utilization is substantially higher in the autumn in the southern region than it is in the northern region.

65 and Over Age Group. It is well known that older people are more susceptible to inclement weather conditions such as severe cold and heat. One would therefore expect evidence of an interaction between weather conditions and age in the utilization statistics pertaining to the 65 and over age group. Such evidence can indeed be deduced from the seasonal patterns of utilization indicators pertaining to this group.

Presented in figures 6-8, 6-9, and 6-10 are the seasonal patterns of admissions for age 65 and over found in three census regions vis-à-vis the national pattern. Notice that in figure 6-8, admissions for age 65 and over in region 5 appear in an exaggerated manner during the summer months. In figures 6-9 and 6-10, fluctuations in admissions for age 65 and over and inpatient days for age 65 and over appear in a somewhat accentuated way: the winter upswings and the summer downswings are more pronounced for the regional indexes than they are for the national indexes.

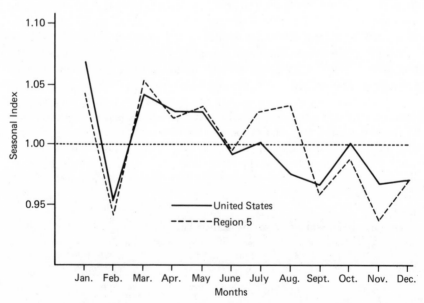

Figure 6-8. Admissions: Age 65 and Over—United States and Region 5 (East South Central)

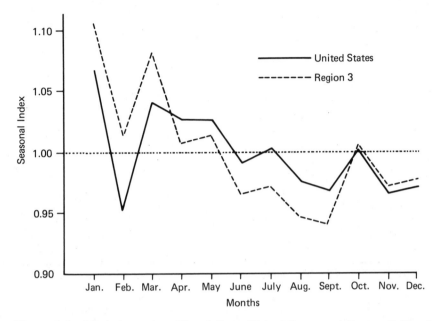

Figure 6-9. Admissions: Age 65 and Over—United States and Region 3 (South Atlantic)

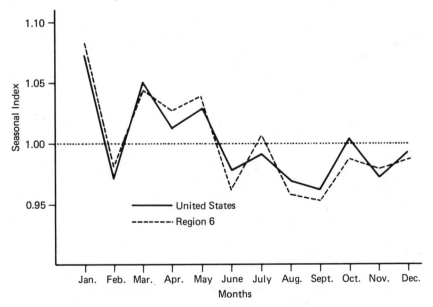

Figure 6-10. Inpatient Days: Age 65 and Over—United States and Region 6 (West North Central)

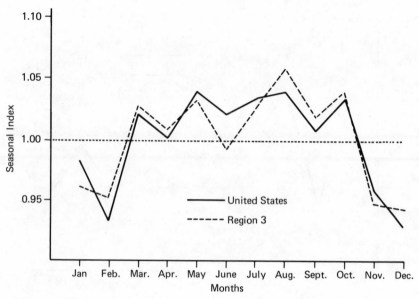

Figure 6-11. Outpatient Visits: United States and Region 3 (South Atlantic)

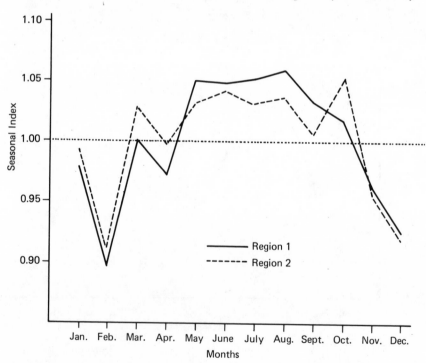

Figure 6-12. Outpatient Visits: Region 1 (New England) and Region 2 (Middle Atlantic)

Type 3 Indicators

The fact that outpatient visits and surgical operations are placed in type 3 does not mean that the general shape or configuration of these indicators change from region to region. It is only when we compare regions that are far apart in terms of climatic conditions does this phenomenon occur, thus underscoring the sensitivity of these indicators to climatic and perhaps topographical and socio-economic variations. Aside from these instances, the seasonal pattern of outpatient visits and surgical operations take on the characteristics of type 2 indicators, with the difference confined to the degree of severity of peaks and troughs.

Outpatient Visits. Displayed in figure 6-11 are the seasonal patterns of the nation and census region 3 (South Atlantic). It is apparent that aside from the exaggerated downswing in June and upswing in August that appear in the regional indexes, the general configuration is substantially the same. Figure 6-12 displays, side by side, the seasonal patterns of two geographically contiguous census regions—region 1 (New England) and region 2 (Middle Atlantic). Here again, the configurations are substantially the same.

Figure 6-13 displays, side by side, the seasonal patterns of two regions which offer the greatest contrast: New England, which comes closest to the

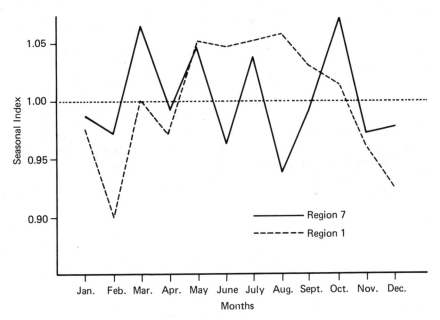

Figure 6-13. Outpatient Visits: Region 1 (New England) and Region 7 (West South Central)

Subfrigid Zone, and West South Central, which comes closest to the Torrid Zone. The differences are striking. The troughs in winter are deeper in New England, presumably because inclement weather severely restricts outdoor activities. Outpatient activity is uniformly high during the summer months in New England. It may be that the New Englanders are more apt to develop "cabin fever" during winter, so they are more disposed to spend more time outdoors in the summer season. The highly urban characteristics of New England may also be a causative factor. High temperatures, when combined with pollutants, produce high ozone levels sending people with respiratory problems to the outpatient departments. The seasonal pattern of region 7, on the other hand, exhibits a high degree of month-to-month fluctuations. Indeed, the graph resembles the jagged edge of a saw. Thus figure 6-13 represents a case where seasonal patterns exhibit configurative differences.

Surgical Operations. Figures 6-14 through 6-16 compare the seasonal patterns of surgical operations in various census regions. Figure 6-14 compares the seasonal pattern observed in region 7 (West South Central) against the national pattern. As can be seen, while there are basic similarities, the summer upswings and the winter downswings of region 7 appear in a highly accentuated form. Figures 6-15 and 6-16 display the seasonal patterns of regions which offer the greatest contrast in terms of climatic zones: region 1 (New England) versus region 5 (East South Central), and region 2 (Middle Atlantic) versus region 7 (West South Central). Notice that both graphs exhibit configurative differences.

A distinctive feature of the southern regions is the sweeping fluctuations in the level of surgical operations: the summer upswings and the winter downswings are substantially greater than those exhibited by the rest of the regions. There seems to be a causal link between climatic conditions and incidences of surgery. What that link is, we do not know. It may also be that factors other than climate, such as style of care, availability of health professionals, and so on, may also be at play. For example, since the southern regions have a relative undersupply of surgeons,[6] presumably more surgery is done by the general practitioner, who may schedule elective surgery more often during a period when there are fewer medical cases.[7] This practice, when added to the traditional patient preference for surgery during the summer months, could intensify the peak that occurs in summer.

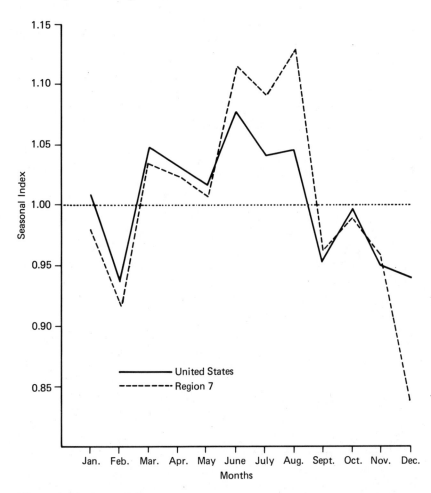

Figure 6-14. Surgical Operations: United States and Region 7 (West South Central)

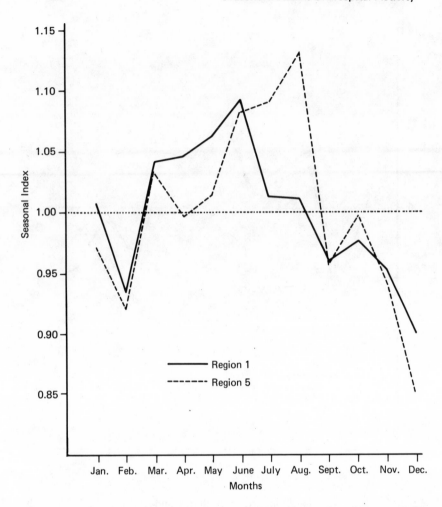

Figure 6-15. Surgical Operations: Region 1 (New England) and Region 5 (East South Central)

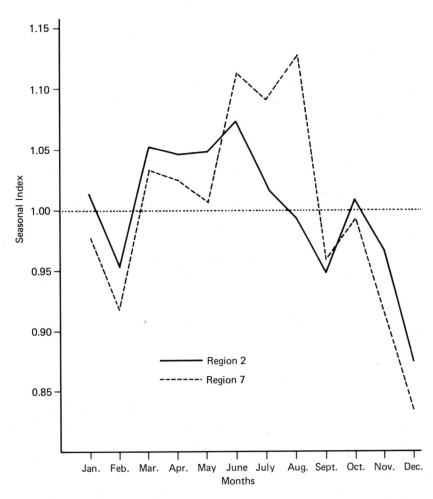

Figure 6-16. Surgical Operations: Region 2 (Middle Atlantic) and Region 7 (West South Central)

Notes

1. A notable exception is census region 9 (Pacific), which includes Alaska and Hawaii.

2. Although this is true in a very broad sense, intraregional differences are likely to be present in those census regions delineated longitudinally. An example is census region 8 (Mountain).

3. According to the 1976 hospital census, Alaska has 15 community hospitals and 766 beds.

4. U.S. Bureau of the Census, *Current Population Reports,* Series P-23, No. 43, U.S. Government Printing Office, Washington, 1973.

5. M. Gornick, "Medicare Patients: Geographic Differences in Hospital Discharge Rates and Multiple Stays," *Social Security Bulletin* (June 1977):28.

6. "College, ASA Release Surgical Study Findings," *Bulletin of the American College of Surgeons* 60 (July 1975):4.

7. Some confirmatory evidence in this regard is provided by analysis of variation *within* region 7. Those states with a relative undersupply of surgeons exhibit demonstrably greater variations in surgical operations while retaining the general shape of the seasonal pattern.

7

Regional Indexes

Regional indexes including a quick reference table of national indexes are provided in tables 7–1 through 7–10. Each row in a table is devoted to an indicator. For example, the first row of table 7–1 presents the seasonal indexes pertaining to inpatient days, the second row presents the seasonal indexes pertaining to admissions, and so on. This format is maintained in tables 7–1 through 7–10.

All indexes are presented in ratio form. It is in this form that the indexes should be used to convert raw values to seasonally adjusted values. It is also customary to express seasonal indexes in percentage form. For instance, instead of expressing an index as 1.0600, we may express it as 106.00. The consumer price index (CPI) is expressed this way. The merit of showing an index in percentage form is that its significance is more readily understood by the laypeople. An index value of 106.00, for example, conveys immediately to the reader the notion that the index is 6 percent above the average (if it is a seasonal index) or 6 percent above the base period value (if it is a price index such as the CPI).

Those interested in national indicators should, of course, consult table 7–1. Those interested in indicators at the regional, state, metropolitan area, or individual hospital level should consult the appropriate regional tables. See figure 7–1 for a description of census regions (divisions).

Table 7–11 displays the measures of amplitude (*MA*). Each column of this table indicates the relative month-to-month fluctuations of various hospital indicators. Perhaps the best way to understand the significance of these values is to refer to a specific *MA* in column 1 of table 7–11 and then refer back to the corresponding graph in chapter 5. For example, column 1 of table 7–11 shows that the measure of amplitude is lowest for beds (*MA* = 0.002). Referring to figure 5–14, we notice that the graph pertaining to beds looks almost like a straight line, with minimal month-to-month variations. In contrast, consider the graph of surgical operations presented in figure 5–19, which has the largest measure of amplitude (*MA* = 0.054). That graph exhibits the widest month-to-month fluctuations. Thus the measures of amplitude presented in table 7–1 provide a handy way of assessing the relative fluctuations of indicators.

Each row of table 7–11 indicates the monthly fluctuations of an indicator in various regions of the United States. For example, the first row of the table shows that monthly fluctuations of inpatient days are the lowest in region 9 (*MA* = 0.031) and the highest in region 8 (*MA* = 0.049).

Table 7-1
Monthly (Seasonal) Indexes: National

	Jan.	Feb.	Mar.	Apr.	May	June	July	Aug.	Sept.	Oct.	Nov.	Dec.
Inpatient days	1.0666	0.9881	1.0624	1.0060	1.0162	0.9774	0.9874	0.9864	0.9629	1.0168	0.9827	0.9471
Admissions	1.0490	0.9571	1.0451	1.0111	1.0039	1.0164	1.0177	1.0228	0.9700	1.0058	0.9643	0.9370
Adjusted admissions	1.0412	0.9538	1.0411	1.0101	1.0053	1.0187	1.0194	1.0286	0.9749	1.0050	0.9643	0.9377
Adjusted patient days	1.0596	0.9840	1.0595	1.0054	1.0176	0.9802	0.9901	0.9909	0.9658	1.0170	0.9825	0.9474
Adult length of stay	1.0185	1.0315	1.0128	0.9939	1.0173	0.9632	0.9693	0.9633	0.9903	1.0092	1.0175	1.0134
Adult daily census	1.0470	1.0635	1.0430	1.0203	0.9974	0.9915	0.9689	0.9681	0.9765	0.9976	0.9965	0.9297
Beds	1.0029	1.0025	1.0015	1.0008	1.0003	0.9983	0.9989	0.9983	0.9986	0.9993	0.9986	1.0001
Occupancy rate	1.0436	1.0609	1.0414	1.0189	0.9974	0.9928	0.9703	0.9702	0.9791	0.9987	0.9977	0.9292
Births	0.9803	0.9175	0.9949	0.9374	0.9739	0.9710	1.0562	1.0719	1.0588	1.0402	0.9823	1.0158
Newborn days	0.9980	0.9267	0.9976	0.9371	0.9762	0.9694	1.0470	1.0638	1.0456	1.0504	0.9858	1.0024
Newborn length of stay	1.0136	1.0115	1.0114	1.0117	1.0122	0.9946	0.9882	0.9882	0.9657	1.0112	1.0035	0.9882
Newborn occupancy rate	0.9856	0.9988	0.9757	0.9534	0.9585	0.9805	1.0283	1.0408	1.0589	1.0320	0.9999	0.9878
Admissions: age 65 and over	1.0695	0.9540	1.0408	1.0265	1.0281	0.9922	1.0027	0.9766	0.9679	1.0030	0.9682	0.9705
Inpatient days: age 65 and over	1.0709	0.9709	1.0500	1.0131	1.0283	0.9768	0.9905	0.9691	0.9619	1.0036	0.9741	0.9910
Length of stay: age 65 and over	0.9998	1.0155	1.0079	0.9875	1.0018	0.9791	0.9893	0.9935	0.9968	1.0008	1.0082	1.0196
Surgical operations	1.0074	0.9470	1.0475	1.0302	1.0161	1.0763	1.0414	1.0454	0.9523	0.9948	0.9517	0.8899
Outpatient visits	0.9831	0.9328	1.0214	1.0001	1.0390	1.0206	1.0335	1.0398	1.0089	1.0347	0.9566	0.9296
Total revenue	1.0425	0.9759	1.0557	1.0045	1.0172	0.9911	0.9956	0.9944	0.9705	1.0164	0.9745	0.9618
Revenue per adjusted patient day	0.9840	0.9908	0.9964	0.9980	0.9989	1.0122	1.0065	1.0011	1.0057	0.9985	0.9918	1.0162
Revenue per adjusted admission	0.9985	1.0214	1.0118	0.9955	1.0109	0.9732	0.9769	0.9661	0.9957	1.0134	1.0093	1.0274
Total expenses	1.0102	0.9611	1.0245	0.9921	1.0061	1.0040	1.0151	1.0102	0.9844	1.0053	0.9798	1.0073
Adjusted expenses per inpatient day	0.9528	0.9760	0.9667	0.9856	0.9865	1.0244	1.0252	1.0165	1.0187	0.9879	0.9960	1.0638
Adjusted expenses per admission	0.9685	1.0066	0.9819	0.9830	0.9990	0.9847	0.9957	0.9802	1.0106	0.9997	1.0155	1.0747

Table 7-2
Monthly (Seasonal) Indexes: Region 1 (New England)

	Jan.	Feb.	Mar.	Apr.	May	June	July	Aug.	Sept.	Oct.	Nov.	Dec.
Inpatient days	1.0666	0.9707	1.0498	1.0097	1.0281	0.9963	0.9688	0.9716	0.9620	1.0203	0.9875	0.9687
Admissions	1.0465	0.9415	1.0322	1.0219	1.0249	1.0306	0.9950	0.9929	0.9776	1.0101	0.9726	0.9543
Adjusted admissions	1.0418	0.9389	1.0313	1.0200	1.0261	1.0327	0.9973	0.9997	0.9842	1.0048	0.9712	0.9519
Adjusted patient days	1.0632	0.9662	1.0485	1.0081	1.0297	1.0001	0.9713	0.9775	0.9683	1.0160	0.9844	0.9668
Adult length of stay	1.0172	1.0357	1.0242	0.9868	0.9986	0.9673	0.9729	0.9742	0.9850	1.0078	1.0147	1.0157
Adult daily census	1.0471	1.0443	1.0307	1.0241	1.0088	1.0108	0.9507	0.9535	0.9759	1.0014	1.0017	0.9510
Beds	1.0045	1.0016	1.0025	1.0036	1.0008	1.0039	0.9952	0.9981	1.0003	0.9924	0.9992	0.9979
Occupancy rate	1.0437	1.0428	1.0285	1.0204	1.0085	1.0054	0.9559	0.9580	0.9752	1.0080	1.0028	0.9510
Births	0.9720	0.9334	1.0300	0.9763	1.0134	0.9967	1.0519	1.0512	1.0287	0.9892	0.9662	0.9909
Newborn days	0.9998	0.9480	1.0451	0.9704	1.0098	1.0023	1.0444	1.0346	1.0076	0.9977	0.9652	0.9753
Newborn length of stay	1.0217	1.0142	1.0079	0.9943	1.0003	1.0057	0.9904	0.9828	0.9791	1.0150	1.0003	0.9884
Newborn occupancy rate	0.9887	1.0221	1.0162	0.9795	0.9815	1.0023	1.0230	1.0022	1.0194	0.9978	0.9922	0.9753
Admissions: age 65 and over	1.0279	0.9191	0.9989	1.0045	1.0486	1.0077	1.0061	0.9876	1.0204	1.0081	1.0024	0.9689
Inpatient days: age 65 and over	1.0415	0.9250	1.0290	0.9989	1.0389	0.9965	0.9918	0.9777	0.9901	1.0358	0.9890	0.9858
Length of stay: age 65 and over	1.0027	1.0091	1.0249	0.9893	0.9903	0.9854	0.9868	0.9943	0.9775	1.0255	0.9951	1.0191
Surgical operations	1.0082	0.9350	1.0426	1.0457	1.0612	1.0914	1.0141	1.0103	0.9612	0.9767	0.9526	0.9009
Outpatient visits	0.9787	0.8998	1.0001	0.9739	1.0503	1.0488	1.0521	1.0592	1.0322	1.0167	0.9633	0.9251
Total revenue	1.0619	0.9758	1.0636	1.0041	1.0283	1.0203	0.9845	0.9640	0.9399	0.9851	0.9701	1.0026
Revenue per adjusted patient day	1.0019	1.0079	1.0151	0.9992	1.0001	1.0165	1.0130	0.9843	0.9709	0.9691	0.9847	1.0375
Revenue per adjusted admission	1.0194	1.0433	1.0330	0.9860	1.0023	0.9828	0.9876	0.9614	0.9556	0.9783	0.9998	1.0506
Total expenses	1.0442	0.9720	1.0476	0.9911	1.0111	1.0308	1.0141	0.9880	0.9483	0.9568	0.9753	1.0208
Adjusted expenses per inpatient day	0.9814	1.0054	0.9978	0.9826	0.9821	1.0302	1.0425	1.0111	0.9792	0.9404	0.9890	1.0585
Adjusted expenses per admission	1.0002	1.0363	1.0166	0.9735	0.9858	0.9969	1.0143	0.9868	0.9620	0.9485	1.0041	1.0749

Table 7-3
Monthly (Seasonal) Indexes: Region 2 (Middle Atlantic)

	Jan.	Feb.	Mar.	Apr.	May	June	July	Aug.	Sept.	Oct.	Nov.	Dec.
Inpatient days	1.0549	0.9746	1.0574	1.0065	1.0329	0.9869	0.9797	0.9778	0.9608	1.0311	0.9888	0.9488
Admissions	1.0416	0.9464	1.0461	1.0209	1.0303	1.0222	1.0088	1.0020	0.9656	1.0163	0.9699	0.9298
Adjusted admissions	1.0364	0.9427	1.0421	1.0218	1.0280	1.0249	1.0107	1.0082	0.9691	1.0164	0.9678	0.9320
Adjusted patient days	1.0500	0.9703	1.0528	1.0066	1.0308	0.9892	0.9832	0.9832	0.9644	1.0306	0.9878	0.9512
Adult length of stay	1.0106	1.0305	1.0112	0.9834	1.0036	0.9668	0.9703	0.9757	0.9958	1.0127	1.0173	1.0222
Adult daily census	1.0354	1.0485	1.0382	1.0208	1.0141	1.0010	0.9616	0.9597	0.9745	1.0118	1.0031	0.9315
Beds	1.0013	1.0020	1.0012	0.9996	1.0003	0.9965	0.9980	0.9974	0.9999	1.0014	1.0002	1.0024
Occupancy rate	1.0345	1.0462	1.0371	1.0219	1.0141	1.0048	0.9629	0.9617	0.9752	1.0098	1.0037	0.9283
Births	0.9738	0.9203	0.9992	0.9538	0.9933	0.9881	1.0565	1.0591	1.0427	1.0419	0.9742	0.9970
Newborn days	0.9901	0.9275	1.0003	0.9520	0.9966	0.9828	1.0427	1.0610	1.0341	1.0489	0.9748	0.9892
Newborn length of stay	1.0139	1.0065	0.9989	0.9986	1.0114	0.9931	0.9892	1.0006	0.9875	1.0086	1.0027	0.9890
Newborn occupancy rate	0.9762	1.0020	0.9812	0.9695	0.9764	0.9984	1.0262	1.0391	1.0471	1.0280	0.9849	0.9711
Admissions: age 65 and over	1.0300	0.9197	1.0265	1.0356	1.0402	1.0102	1.0066	0.9715	0.9764	1.0330	0.9750	0.9754
Inpatient days: age 65 and over	1.0332	0.9414	1.0304	1.0066	1.0411	1.0017	1.0026	0.9707	0.9702	1.0223	0.9868	0.9933
Length of stay: age 65 and over	0.9983	1.0198	1.0063	0.9709	0.9953	0.9857	0.9994	1.0049	0.9952	0.9962	1.0101	1.0181
Surgical operations	1.0130	0.9533	1.0533	1.0454	1.0476	1.0741	1.0185	0.9936	0.9502	1.0082	0.9654	0.8776
Outpatient visits	0.9921	0.9100	1.0265	0.9959	1.0317	1.0422	1.0311	1.0352	1.0051	1.0510	0.9578	0.9216
Total revenue	1.0210	0.9536	1.0423	0.9979	1.0247	0.9998	1.0023	0.9964	0.9827	1.0368	0.9727	0.9698
Revenue per adjusted patient day	0.9723	0.9827	0.9910	0.9901	0.9935	1.0109	1.0181	1.0124	1.0201	1.0048	0.9853	1.0188
Revenue per adjusted admission	0.9844	1.0094	1.0037	0.9769	0.9974	0.9740	0.9890	0.9865	1.0126	1.0198	1.0066	1.0399
Total expenses	0.9935	0.9438	1.0149	0.9853	1.0081	1.0004	1.0231	1.0213	0.9910	1.0236	0.9807	1.0142
Adjusted expenses per inpatient day	0.9450	0.9714	0.9647	0.9771	0.9772	1.0117	1.0403	1.0368	1.0276	0.9911	0.9916	1.0657
Adjusted expenses per admission	0.9565	0.9995	0.9754	0.9643	0.9797	0.9752	1.0138	1.0118	1.0200	1.0054	1.0114	1.0868

Table 7-4
Monthly (Seasonal) Indexes: Region 3 (South Atlantic)

	Jan.	Feb.	Mar.	Apr.	May	June	July	°Aug.	Sept.	Oct.	Nov.	Dec.
Inpatient days	1.0660	1.0016	1.0750	1.0043	1.0122	0.9678	0.9823	0.9856	0.9656	1.0176	0.9865	0.9356
Admissions	1.0480	0.9706	1.0462	0.9986	0.9969	1.0012	1.0197	1.0289	0.9790	1.0047	0.9723	0.9339
Adjusted admissions	1.0386	0.9657	1.0432	0.9968	0.9999	1.0040	1.0226	1.0356	0.9820	1.0075	0.9714	0.9327
Adjusted patient days	1.0572	0.9960	1.0710	1.0032	1.0145	0.9714	0.9853	0.9915	0.9680	1.0203	0.9866	0.9350
Adult length of stay	1.0181	1.0281	1.0219	1.0060	1.0120	0.9659	0.9635	0.9610	0.9842	1.0160	1.0197	1.0037
Adult daily census	1.0461	1.0767	1.0551	1.0188	0.9935	0.9818	0.9638	0.9672	0.9795	0.9986	1.0004	0.9184
Beds	0.9997	1.0011	1.0028	1.0015	0.9991	1.0032	0.9987	0.9981	0.9966	1.0006	1.0004	0.9981
Occupancy rate	1.0452	1.0765	1.0520	1.0162	0.9946	0.9783	0.9654	0.9697	0.9838	0.9981	1.0003	0.9199
Births	1.0048	0.9354	0.9875	0.9146	0.9433	0.9342	1.0364	1.0727	1.0746	1.0431	0.9972	1.0561
Newborn days	1.0137	0.9396	0.9874	0.9143	0.9424	0.9311	1.0376	1.0777	1.0561	1.0566	1.0062	1.0373
Newborn length of stay	1.0136	1.0040	0.9982	0.9960	0.9916	0.9937	1.0160	0.9984	0.9873	1.0167	1.0025	0.9822
Newborn occupancy rate	0.9911	1.0216	0.9619	0.9346	0.9296	0.9475	1.0065	1.0506	1.0702	1.0459	1.0218	1.0186
Admissions: age 65 and over	1.1066	1.0130	1.0815	1.0072	1.0137	0.9651	0.9725	0.9464	0.9400	1.0055	0.9702	0.9783
Inpatient days: age 65 and over	1.0892	1.0074	1.0859	1.0107	1.0222	0.9641	0.9621	0.9437	0.9303	1.0115	0.9818	0.9913
Length of stay: age 65 and over	0.9810	0.9902	1.0080	0.9991	1.0050	1.0005	0.9942	0.9999	0.9886	1.0078	1.0142	1.0114
Surgical operations	0.9947	0.9476	1.0416	1.0165	1.0159	1.0595	1.0512	1.0665	0.9719	1.0105	0.9557	0.8685
Outpatient visits	0.9617	0.9513	1.0266	1.0067	1.0322	0.9901	1.0270	1.0578	1.0177	1.0388	0.9483	0.9419
Total revenue	1.0501	0.9910	1.0676	1.0110	1.0089	0.9817	0.9810	0.9846	0.9706	1.0140	0.9770	0.9627
Revenue per adjusted patient day	0.9941	0.9932	0.9958	1.0079	0.9927	1.0078	0.9941	0.9930	1.0027	0.9977	0.9896	1.0313
Revenue per adjusted admission	1.0108	1.0211	1.0213	1.0153	1.0073	0.9749	0.9603	0.9536	0.9849	1.0132	1.0057	1.0316
Total expenses	1.0089	0.9696	1.0200	0.9934	1.0022	1.0071	0.9934	1.0023	0.9870	1.0095	0.9906	1.0162
Adjusted expenses per inpatient day	0.9541	0.9710	0.9505	0.9880	0.9844	1.0363	1.0070	1.0095	1.0178	0.9919	1.0008	1.0885
Adjusted expenses per admission	0.9701	1.0006	0.9741	0.9967	0.9986	1.0036	0.9699	0.9675	1.0032	1.0068	1.0173	1.0915

Table 7-5
Monthly (Seasonal) Indexes: Region 4 (East North Central)

	Jan.	Feb.	Mar.	Apr.	May	June	July	Aug.	Sept.	Oct.	Nov.	Dec.
Inpatient days	1.0606	0.9846	1.0541	1.0043	1.0192	0.9789	0.9873	0.9867	0.9663	1.0213	0.9873	0.9495
Admissions	1.0423	0.9501	1.0402	1.0141	1.0062	1.0223	1.0152	1.0179	0.9737	1.0139	0.9674	0.9368
Adjusted admissions	1.0343	0.9454	1.0373	1.0133	1.0102	1.0272	1.0177	1.0226	0.9775	1.0157	0.9659	0.9332
Adjusted patient days	1.0526	0.9802	1.0509	1.0033	1.0218	0.9832	0.9900	0.9930	0.9703	1.0221	0.9861	0.9466
Adult length of stay	1.0152	1.0358	1.0169	0.9890	1.0101	0.9581	0.9713	0.9711	0.9923	1.0100	1.0190	1.0113
Adult daily census	1.0411	1.0580	1.0350	1.0184	1.0004	0.9930	0.9687	0.9686	0.9803	1.0028	1.0017	0.9321
Beds	1.0031	1.0028	1.0025	1.0013	1.0017	0.9986	0.9979	0.9958	0.9970	1.0010	0.9987	0.9996
Occupancy rate	1.0384	1.0557	1.0326	1.0160	0.9986	0.9945	0.9709	0.9735	0.9834	1.0027	1.0023	0.9314
Births	0.9769	0.9146	0.9962	0.9456	0.9872	0.9906	1.0564	1.0550	1.0481	1.0370	0.9828	1.0096
Newborn days	1.0013	0.9236	0.9987	0.9454	0.9893	0.9809	1.0451	1.0500	1.0403	1.0422	0.9837	0.9998
Newborn length of stay	1.0179	1.0081	1.0083	1.0037	1.0041	0.9796	0.9799	1.0037	0.9905	1.0060	1.0092	0.9890
Newbory occupancy rate	0.9774	0.9932	0.9784	0.9621	0.9711	0.9931	1.0312	1.0365	1.0565	1.0193	0.9997	0.9815
Admissions: age 65 and over	1.0461	0.9210	1.0251	1.0222	1.0435	1.0049	1.0126	0.9876	0.9824	1.0163	0.9711	0.9673
Inpatient days: age 65 and over	1.0557	0.9514	1.0240	1.0045	1.0389	0.9821	1.0029	0.9845	0.9741	1.0030	0.9762	1.0029
Length of stay: age 65 and over	1.0061	1.0331	0.9985	0.9788	0.9934	0.9741	0.9935	0.9935	0.9957	0.9917	1.0062	1.0355
Surgical operations	1.0151	0.9598	1.0471	1.0290	1.0121	1.0784	1.0261	1.0350	0.9423	0.9998	0.9488	0.9064
Outpatient visits	0.9668	0.9149	1.0163	0.9946	1.0405	1.0466	1.0522	1.0555	1.0231	1.0405	0.9427	0.9063
Total revenue	1.0386	0.9761	1.0461	1.0034	1.0239	0.9954	0.9964	0.9942	0.9695	1.0158	0.9775	0.9630
Revenue per adjusted patient day	0.9867	0.9967	0.9946	0.9991	0.9992	1.0138	1.0066	1.0009	0.9979	0.9936	0.9927	1.0182
Revenue per adjusted admission	1.0025	1.0304	1.0083	0.9907	1.0106	0.9693	0.9802	0.9694	0.9937	1.0028	1.0118	1.0303
Total expenses	1.0114	0.9546	1.0233	0.9893	1.0062	1.0040	1.0194	1.0040	0.9882	1.0073	0.9819	1.0104
Adjusted expenses per inpatient day	0.9605	0.9726	0.9713	0.9849	0.9827	1.0216	1.0285	1.0116	1.0184	0.9854	0.9956	1.0670
Adjusted expenses per admission	0.9771	1.0076	0.9860	0.9760	0.9942	0.9764	1.0012	0.9809	1.0112	0.9918	1.0160	1.0816

Table 7-6
Monthly (Seasonal) Indexes: Region 5 (East South Central)

	Jan.	Feb.	Mar.	Apr.	May	June	July	Aug.	Sept.	Oct.	Nov.	Dec.
Inpatient days	1.0618	0.9944	1.0689	0.9952	1.0106	0.9775	0.9958	1.0150	0.9726	1.0154	0.9672	0.9258
Admissions	1.0376	0.9523	1.0399	0.9889	0.9928	1.0100	1.0399	1.0683	0.9853	1.0040	0.9526	0.9284
Adjusted admissions	1.0295	0.9397	1.0417	0.9906	0.9990	1.0087	1.0480	1.0761	0.9874	1.0044	0.9498	0.9253
Adjusted patient days	1.0496	0.9830	1.0700	0.9962	1.0148	0.9792	1.0016	1.0272	0.9749	1.0139	0.9650	0.9247
Adult length of stay	1.0223	1.0414	1.0272	1.0030	1.0168	0.9669	0.9585	0.9522	0.9885	1.0069	1.0196	0.9967
Adult daily census	1.0425	1.0677	1.0490	1.0097	0.9923	0.9918	0.9773	0.9965	0.9867	0.9967	0.9813	0.9084
Beds	1.0011	1.0011	1.0012	1.0010	1.0031	0.9981	1.0020	0.9983	0.9975	0.9988	0.9987	0.9992
Occupancy rate	1.0410	1.0665	1.0472	1.0074	0.9886	0.9941	0.9764	0.9996	0.9893	0.9967	0.9836	0.9096
Births	0.9987	0.8870	0.9655	0.9009	0.9075	0.9372	1.0728	1.1092	1.0820	1.0797	1.0102	1.0495
Newborn days	1.0047	0.8880	0.9745	0.8944	0.9116	0.9193	1.0673	1.1042	1.0670	1.1073	1.0270	1.0349
Newborn length of stay	1.0115	1.0069	1.0011	0.9938	1.0028	0.9765	0.9918	0.9919	0.9871	1.0216	1.0279	0.9872
Newborn occupancy rate	1.0017	0.9706	0.9535	0.9113	0.9074	0.9330	1.0354	1.0776	1.0838	1.0790	1.0357	1.0113
Admissions: age 65 and over	1.0431	0.9446	1.0529	1.0212	1.0290	0.9939	1.0271	1.0339	0.9581	0.9868	0.9393	0.9702
Inpatient days: age 65 and over	1.0732	0.9737	1.0612	1.0224	1.0341	0.9761	0.9888	1.0034	0.9546	0.9935	0.9519	0.9671
Length of stay: age 65 and over	1.0263	1.0264	1.0066	0.9990	1.0023	0.9848	0.9612	0.9681	0.9981	1.0088	1.0207	0.9978
Surgical operations	0.9702	0.9204	1.0356	0.9970	1.0150	1.0869	1.0928	1.1329	0.9587	0.9978	0.9412	0.8516
Outpatient visits	0.9728	0.9226	1.0263	1.0213	1.0239	0.9649	1.0486	1.0684	1.0261	1.0175	0.9755	0.9323
Total revenue	1.0405	0.9765	1.0656	1.0031	1.0094	0.9906	1.0079	1.0189	0.9975	0.9953	0.9696	0.9251
Revenue per adjusted patient day	0.9889	0.9932	0.9988	1.0082	0.9983	1.0118	1.0000	0.9917	1.0203	0.9835	1.0039	1.0016
Revenue per adjusted admission	1.0092	1.0356	1.0221	1.0162	1.0111	0.9808	0.9563	0.9455	1.0097	0.9920	1.0207	1.0009
Total expenses	1.0110	0.9634	1.0238	0.9959	1.0049	1.0061	1.0157	1.0145	0.9893	1.0044	0.9785	0.9927
Adjusted expenses per inpatient day	0.9604	0.9772	0.9562	0.9991	0.9906	1.0284	1.0103	0.9866	1.0130	0.9906	1.0106	1.0771
Adjusted expenses per admission	0.9827	1.0258	0.9794	1.0071	1.0046	0.9961	0.9663	0.9409	0.9998	0.9975	1.0272	1.0725

Table 7-7
Monthly (Seasonal) Indexes: Region 6 (West North Central)

	Jan.	Feb.	Mar.	Apr.	May	June	July	Aug.	Sept.	Oct.	Nov.	Dec.
Inpatient days	1.0970	1.0069	1.0739	1.0131	1.0058	0.9606	0.9769	0.9729	0.9512	1.0031	0.9801	0.9586
Admissions	1.0830	0.9807	1.0589	1.0189	0.9930	1.0068	0.9976	1.0086	0.9559	0.9916	0.9574	0.9475
Adjusted admissions	1.0754	0.9795	1.0577	1.0178	0.9962	1.0083	1.0000	1.0125	0.9584	0.9933	0.9575	0.9435
Adjusted patient days	1.0902	1.0062	1.0730	1.0125	1.0080	0.9622	0.9791	0.9763	0.9537	1.0038	0.9793	0.9559
Adult length of stay	1.0123	1.0244	1.0139	0.9972	1.0141	0.9560	0.9761	0.9675	0.9939	1.0090	1.0233	1.0125
Adult daily census	1.0770	1.0809	1.0544	1.0275	0.9875	0.9743	0.9589	0.9549	0.9649	0.9845	0.9940	0.9411
Beds	1.0078	1.0064	1.0015	0.9998	1.0012	0.9953	0.9973	0.9962	0.9979	0.9966	0.9975	1.0025
Occupancy rate	1.0681	1.0734	1.0523	1.0273	0.9880	0.9795	0.9615	0.9591	0.9686	0.9886	0.9973	0.9363
Births	0.9645	0.9089	1.0008	0.9350	0.9748	0.9778	1.0668	1.0859	1.0534	1.0454	0.9883	0.9984
Newborn days	0.9909	0.9205	1.0011	0.9389	0.9756	0.9731	1.0615	1.0656	1.0440	1.0472	0.9925	0.9891
Newborn length of stay	1.0146	1.0137	1.0171	1.0116	1.0094	0.9953	0.9976	0.9783	0.9875	0.9918	0.9973	0.9859
Newborn occupancy rate	0.9881	0.9926	0.9851	0.9515	0.9575	0.9832	1.0411	1.0480	1.0605	1.0258	0.9942	0.9724
Admissions: age 65 and over	1.0694	0.9620	1.0389	1.0420	1.0460	0.9875	1.0134	0.9625	0.9578	0.9932	0.9575	0.9698
Inpatient days: age 65 and over	1.0822	0.9791	1.0466	1.0263	1.0356	0.9606	1.0059	0.9585	0.9536	0.9875	0.9765	0.9877
Length of stay: age 65 and over	1.0068	1.0184	1.0043	0.9777	0.9868	0.9731	0.9925	1.0028	0.9971	1.0005	1.0199	1.0202
Surgical operations	1.0501	0.9594	1.0484	1.0204	0.9974	1.0775	1.0301	1.0388	0.9343	0.9774	0.9514	0.9147
Outpatient visits	0.9666	0.9304	1.0052	1.0089	1.0380	1.0112	1.0428	1.0546	0.9968	1.0445	0.9641	0.9367
Total revenue	1.0723	1.0056	1.0624	1.0174	1.0132	0.9633	0.9911	0.9907	0.9633	1.0030	0.9684	0.9493
Revenue per adjusted patient day	0.9869	1.0004	0.9910	1.0039	1.0004	1.0004	1.0124	1.0122	1.0101	1.0008	0.9873	0.9943
Revenue per adjusted admission	1.0019	1.0243	1.0044	0.9994	1.0153	0.9582	0.9884	0.9791	1.0054	1.0073	1.0084	1.0080
Total expenses	1.0211	0.9718	1.0260	0.9985	1.0116	0.9854	1.0182	1.0119	0.9862	0.9965	0.9722	1.0006
Adjusted expenses per inpatient day	0.9384	0.9667	0.9556	0.9841	1.0011	1.0215	1.0388	1.0314	1.0316	0.9941	0.9896	1.0472
Adjusted expenses per admission	0.9528	0.9929	0.9703	0.9784	1.0133	0.9746	1.0156	0.9982	1.0298	1.0022	1.0127	1.0593

Table 7-8
Monthly (Seasonal) Indexes: Region 7 (West South Central)

	Jan.	Feb.	Mar.	Apr.	May	June	July	Aug.	Sept.	Oct.	Nov.	Dec.
Inpatient days	1.0802	0.9982	1.0604	0.9935	1.0002	0.9805	1.0135	1.0126	0.9712	1.0067	0.9645	0.9186
Admissions	1.0686	0.9647	1.0433	0.9935	0.9893	1.0160	1.0394	1.0561	0.9725	0.9945	0.9469	0.9151
Adjusted admissions	1.0638	0.9642	1.0426	0.9942	0.9904	1.0160	1.0428	1.0585	0.9691	0.9934	0.9458	0.9192
Adjusted patient days	1.0748	0.9952	1.0572	0.9953	1.0008	0.9798	1.0184	1.0131	0.9715	1.0065	0.9656	0.9220
Adult length of stay	1.0100	1.0317	1.0174	1.0039	1.0081	0.9611	0.9685	0.9617	0.9989	1.0213	1.0165	1.0009
Adult daily census	1.0604	1.0738	1.0410	1.0078	0.9815	0.9946	0.9947	0.9938	0.9848	0.9879	0.9780	0.9017
Beds	0.9984	1.0012	1.0009	0.9991	1.0013	1.0011	1.0002	0.9992	0.9992	1.0035	0.9991	0.9968
Occupancy rate	1.0614	1.0716	1.0399	1.0089	0.9779	0.9928	0.9949	0.9956	0.9863	0.9859	0.9805	0.9042
Births	0.9992	0.9188	0.9582	0.8784	0.9154	0.9421	1.0419	1.1106	1.0933	1.0750	1.0056	1.0616
Newborn days	1.0139	0.9309	0.9555	0.8869	0.9328	0.9467	1.0402	1.0906	1.0718	1.0783	1.0114	1.0412
Newborn length of stay	1.0234	1.0059	1.0034	1.0196	1.0200	0.9989	0.9906	0.9766	0.9753	1.0056	1.0011	0.9794
Newborn occupancy rate	0.9982	0.9867	0.9323	0.8967	0.9137	0.9514	1.0205	1.0709	1.0922	1.0670	1.0376	1.0331
Admissions: age 65 and over	1.0801	0.9781	1.0506	1.0175	0.9979	0.9788	1.0190	1.0107	0.9679	0.9904	0.9484	0.9605
Inpatient days: age 65 and over	1.0956	1.0040	1.0648	1.0019	0.9908	0.9621	0.9954	0.9943	0.9687	0.9896	0.9642	0.9686
Length of stay: age 65 and over	1.0080	1.0238	1.0107	0.9819	1.0010	0.9783	0.9777	0.9814	1.0022	1.0055	1.0163	1.0133
Surgical operations	0.9793	0.9173	1.0344	1.0240	1.0083	1.1137	1.0916	1.1255	0.9575	0.9919	0.9179	0.8387
Outpatient visits	0.9857	0.9701	1.0564	0.9926	1.0457	0.9619	1.0360	0.9388	0.9932	1.0713	0.9702	0.9781
Total revenue	1.0711	0.9719	1.0608	1.0040	0.9993	0.9973	1.0138	1.0060	0.9643	1.0146	0.9639	0.9331
Revenue per adjusted patient day	0.9954	0.9771	1.0031	1.0072	0.9994	1.0193	0.9917	0.9884	0.9963	1.0095	0.9989	1.0138
Revenue per adjusted admission	1.0032	1.0076	1.0155	1.0104	1.0061	0.9821	0.9727	0.9514	0.9957	1.0223	1.0150	1.0182
Total expenses	1.0095	0.9568	1.0219	0.9956	1.0012	1.0150	1.0276	1.0110	0.9896	1.0122	0.9714	0.9884
Adjusted expenses per inpatient day	0.9405	0.9593	0.9636	0.9991	1.0006	1.0384	1.0064	0.9903	1.0188	1.0044	1.0050	1.0739
Adjusted expenses per admission	0.9488	0.9882	0.9789	1.0017	1.0070	1.0002	0.9831	0.9535	1.0221	1.0160	1.0235	1.0770

Table 7–9
Monthly (Seasonal) Indexes: Region 8 (Mountain)

	Jan.	Feb.	Mar.	Apr.	May	June	July	Aug.	Sept.	Oct.	Nov.	Dec.
Inpatient days	1.1000	1.0064	1.0840	1.0232	0.9986	0.9752	0.9764	0.9733	0.9313	0.9948	0.9829	0.9540
Admissions	1.0708	0.9647	1.0603	1.0194	0.9883	1.0243	1.0096	1.0099	0.9380	0.9934	0.9702	0.9511
Adjusted admissions	1.0635	0.9617	1.0550	1.0201	0.9887	1.0283	1.0127	1.0136	0.9384	0.9984	0.9703	0.9493
Adjusted patient days	1.0940	1.0026	1.0784	1.0241	1.0000	0.9787	0.9788	0.9769	0.9336	0.9988	0.9807	0.9533
Adult length of stay	1.0236	1.0430	1.0225	0.9991	1.0084	0.9495	0.9674	0.9647	0.9922	0.9989	1.0248	1.0061
Adult daily census	1.0797	1.0823	1.0638	1.0373	0.9800	0.9892	0.9583	0.9550	0.9446	0.9766	0.9967	0.9365
Beds	1.0076	1.0036	1.0008	1.0040	0.9967	1.0049	1.0002	0.9917	0.9913	0.9944	1.0003	1.0047
Occupancy rate	1.0692	1.0801	1.0632	1.0316	0.9852	0.9839	0.9560	0.9620	0.9510	0.9825	0.9992	0.9361
Births	0.9266	0.9132	1.0186	0.9758	1.0173	0.9820	1.0772	1.0655	1.0252	1.0198	0.9664	1.0125
Newborn days	0.9555	0.9192	1.0258	0.9754	1.0127	0.9759	1.0580	1.0640	1.0194	1.0258	0.9642	1.0043
Newborn length of stay	1.0364	1.0082	1.0027	1.0003	0.9885	0.9908	0.9873	0.9976	0.9934	1.0038	1.0024	0.9887
Newborn occupancy rate	0.9643	0.9948	0.9981	0.9831	0.9896	0.9914	1.0482	1.0392	1.0332	1.0075	0.9690	0.9816
Admissions: age 65 and over	1.0777	0.9844	1.0540	1.0155	0.9869	0.9827	1.0079	0.9563	0.9593	1.0120	1.0007	0.9624
Inpatient days: age 65 and over	1.1297	1.0336	1.0811	1.0236	1.0105	0.9303	0.9610	0.9405	0.9214	0.9887	0.9891	0.9906
Length of stay: age 65 and over	1.0594	1.0369	1.0254	0.9947	1.0207	0.9408	0.9645	0.9828	0.9779	0.9742	0.9860	1.0367
Surgical operations	1.0333	0.9757	1.0637	1.0127	0.9793	1.0717	1.0377	1.0423	0.9319	0.9818	0.9654	0.9046
Outpatient visits	1.0363	0.9432	1.0206	1.0401	1.0616	0.9934	1.0271	1.0150	0.9818	1.0051	0.9657	0.9104
Total revenue	1.0657	0.9969	1.0686	1.0174	1.0263	0.9957	0.9995	0.9833	0.9360	0.9932	0.9706	0.9468
Revenue per adjusted patient day	0.9754	0.9939	0.9939	0.9930	1.0232	1.0181	1.0175	1.0073	1.0052	0.9912	0.9858	0.9954
Revenue per adjusted admission	1.0027	1.0393	1.0162	0.9913	1.0302	0.9720	0.9832	0.9727	0.9955	0.9936	1.0010	1.0024
Total expenses	1.0249	0.9791	1.0295	1.0024	1.0131	1.0121	1.0209	0.9968	0.9681	0.9938	0.9791	0.9803
Adjusted expenses per inpatient day	0.9371	0.9756	0.9512	0.9810	1.0085	1.0317	1.0384	1.0209	1.0373	0.9967	0.9969	1.0249
Adjusted expenses per admission	0.9638	1.0172	0.9735	0.9841	1.0163	0.9871	1.0055	0.9808	1.0321	0.9977	1.0080	1.0338

Table 7-10
Monthly (Seasonal) Indexes: Region 9 (Pacific)

	Jan.	Feb.	Mar.	Apr.	May	June	July	Aug.	Sept.	Oct.	Nov.	Dec.
Inpatient days	1.0500	0.9857	1.0608	1.0136	1.0096	0.9652	1.0028	0.9941	0.9633	1.0070	0.9809	0.9671
Admissions	1.0401	0.9603	1.0477	1.0209	0.9929	1.0126	1.0258	1.0250	0.9700	0.9908	0.9621	0.9519
Adjusted admissions	1.0390	0.9593	1.0487	1.0220	0.9968	1.0140	1.0232	1.0268	0.9703	0.9910	0.9582	0.9508
Adjusted patient days	1.0493	0.9849	1.0594	1.0136	1.0127	0.9677	1.0012	0.9959	0.9634	1.0071	0.9779	0.9669
Adult length of stay	1.0100	1.0248	1.0127	0.9921	1.0207	0.9519	0.9727	0.9717	0.9894	1.0140	1.0253	1.0147
Adult daily census	1.0310	1.0580	1.0415	1.0283	0.9911	0.9794	0.9843	0.9760	0.9775	0.9884	0.9949	0.9497
Beds	1.0024	1.0020	0.9983	1.0002	0.9963	0.9950	1.0007	1.0037	1.0036	0.9989	0.9991	1.0000
Occupancy rate	1.0306	1.0565	1.0440	1.0265	0.9933	0.9856	0.9831	0.9695	0.9755	0.9893	0.9973	0.9490
Births	0.9604	0.9021	1.0037	0.9672	1.0100	0.9922	1.0644	1.0669	1.0571	1.0101	0.9579	1.0079
Newborn days	0.9791	0.9218	1.0060	0.9616	1.0101	0.9845	1.0539	1.0614	1.0470	1.0210	0.9620	0.9917
Newborn length of stay	1.0355	1.0242	0.9919	0.9838	0.9903	0.9846	0.9897	0.9918	0.9892	1.0191	1.0182	0.9817
Newborn occupancy rate	0.9700	0.9863	0.9940	0.9808	0.9865	0.9969	1.0416	1.0379	1.0603	1.0004	0.9737	0.9716
Admissions: age 65 and over	1.0948	0.9731	1.0380	1.0227	1.0111	0.9779	0.9995	0.9574	0.9688	0.9928	0.9829	0.9812
Inpatient days: age 65 and over	1.0959	0.9939	1.0534	1.0065	1.0067	0.9619	0.9904	0.9577	0.9774	0.9940	0.9632	0.9990
Length of stay: age 65 and over	0.9990	1.0126	1.0110	0.9731	0.9917	0.9773	1.0003	1.0114	1.0098	0.9972	0.9970	1.0199
Surgical operations	1.0038	0.9515	1.0557	1.0490	0.9848	1.0502	1.0493	1.0488	0.9582	0.9721	0.9590	0.9176
Outpatient visits	0.9972	0.9669	1.0296	1.0088	1.0510	1.0205	1.0045	1.0305	0.9881	1.0044	0.9557	0.9428
Total revenue	1.0271	0.9774	1.0576	1.0099	1.0075	0.9773	1.0012	1.0056	0.9733	1.0142	0.9727	0.9761
Revenue per adjusted patient day	0.9803	0.9943	0.9948	0.9955	0.9984	1.0132	0.9970	1.0102	1.0077	1.0058	0.9934	1.0094
Revenue per adjusted admission	0.9886	1.0216	1.0029	0.9864	1.0131	0.9665	0.9753	0.9799	1.0056	1.0201	1.0143	1.0257
Total expenses	1.0061	0.9727	1.0325	0.9950	1.0063	0.9938	1.0061	1.0174	0.9859	1.0027	0.9765	1.0050
Adjusted expenses per inpatient day	0.9568	0.9869	0.9711	0.9822	0.9932	1.0299	1.0040	1.0241	1.0212	0.9939	0.9977	1.0390
Adjusted expenses per admission	0.9631	1.0148	0.9809	0.9759	1.0111	0.9825	0.9806	0.9920	1.0170	1.0115	1.0166	1.0540

Table 7-11
Measures of Amplitude (MA): United States and Census Regions

Indicator	U.S. National	Region 1 (New England)	Region 2 (Middle Atlantic)	Region 3 (South Atlantic)	Region 4 (East North Central)	Region 5 (East South Central)	Region 6 (West North Central)	Region 7 (West South Central)	Region 8 (Mountain)	Region 9 (Pacific)
Inpatient days	0.036	0.035	0.036	0.040	0.033	0.039	0.045	0.042	0.049	0.031
Admissions	0.035	0.033	0.038	0.033	0.035	0.042	0.040	0.046	0.041	0.033
Adjusted admissions	0.034	0.033	0.037	0.033	0.035	0.046	0.039	0.046	0.040	0.034
Adjusted patient days	0.034	0.034	0.034	0.038	0.032	0.039	0.043	0.040	0.047	0.031
Adult length of stay	0.024	0.022	0.021	0.025	0.024	0.028	0.022	0.024	0.028	0.024
Adult daily census	0.038	0.035	0.036	0.044	0.035	0.041	0.048	0.045	0.053	0.032
Beds	0.002	0.004	0.002	0.002	0.002	0.002	0.004	0.002	0.005	0.003
Occupancy rate	0.037	0.033	0.036	0.043	0.034	0.040	0.045	0.044	0.049	0.032
Births	0.049	0.036	0.043	0.058	0.044	0.079	0.054	0.077	0.050	0.049
Newborn days	0.045	0.031	0.040	0.056	0.040	0.081	0.047	0.067	0.043	0.042
Newborn length of stay	0.015	0.013	0.009	0.011	0.012	0.015	0.013	0.017	0.013	0.019
Newborn occupancy rate	0.033	0.017	0.028	0.047	0.029	0.065	0.036	0.065	0.027	0.030
Admissions: age 65 and over	0.035	0.032	0.037	0.051	0.036	0.040	0.040	0.038	0.037	0.038
Inpatient days: age 65 and over	0.036	0.033	0.030	0.050	0.029	0.040	0.040	0.041	0.062	0.040
Length of stay: age 65 and over	0.012	0.016	0.013	0.010	0.019	0.021	0.016	0.016	0.035	0.014
Surgical operations	0.055	0.056	0.056	0.058	0.050	0.080	0.052	0.086	0.052	0.049
Outpatient visits	0.041	0.053	0.047	0.040	0.054	0.046	0.042	0.042	0.044	0.032
Total revenue	0.029	0.038	0.028	0.032	0.027	0.035	0.038	0.039	0.041	0.026
Revenue per adjusted patient day	0.009	0.020	0.016	0.012	0.009	0.010	0.009	0.012	0.014	0.009
Revenue per adjusted admission	0.019	0.031	0.019	0.025	0.020	0.027	0.018	0.021	0.021	0.020
Total expenses	0.018	0.033	0.023	0.014	0.019	0.017	0.018	0.021	0.020	0.017
Adjusted expenses per inpatient day	0.031	0.032	0.036	0.037	0.030	0.032	0.035	0.036	0.033	0.025
Adjusted expenses per admission	0.027	0.034	0.035	0.033	0.029	0.033	0.029	0.034	0.023	0.025

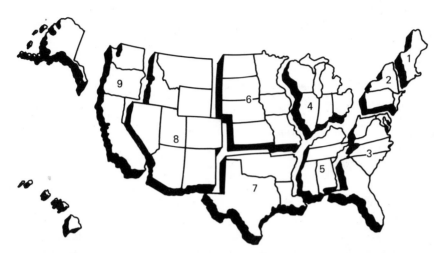

1. New England
    Connecticut
    Maine
    Massachusetts
    New Hampshire
    Rhode Island
    Vermont

2. Middle Atlantic
    Pennsylvania
    New Jersey
    New York

3. South Atlantic
    Delaware
    District of Columbia
    Florida
    Georgia
    Maryland
    North Carolina
    South Carolina
    Virginia
    West Virginia

4. East North Central
    Illinois
    Indiana
    Michigan
    Ohio
    Wisconsin

5. East South Central
    Alabama
    Kentucky
    Mississippi
    Tennessee

6. West North Central
    Iowa
    Kansas
    Minnesota
    Missouri
    Nebraska
    North Dakota
    South Dakota

7. West South Central
    Arkansas
    Louisiana
    Oklahoma
    Texas

8. Mountain
    Arizona
    Colorado
    Idaho
    Montana
    Nevada
    New Mexico
    Utah
    Wyoming

9. Pacific
    Alaska
    California
    Hawaii
    Oregon
    Washington

Source: American Hospital Association, *Selected Community Hospital Indicators, 1976.*
Reprinted with permission.

Figure 7-1. Census Regions

Validity Tests

The indexes developed for a census region are by definition fully applicable to that region as a whole. Are they applicable to the states, metropolitan areas, and individual hospitals belonging to that region? A priori, one must assume that they are. But the vagaries of microdata being what they are, this assumption cannot be taken for granted. We have therefore performed the following validity tests.

There are twenty-three hospital indicators and fifty-one states (including the District of Columbia). Thus the number of all possible tests total 23 × 51 = 1,173. Since this is an enormous undertaking, the validity tests performed were of a limited nature, as shown below:

Number of States/ Hospitals Tested	Number of Indicators Tested	Number of Months Tested
9 states	20	5
18 hospitals	9	12

One state was selected at random from each of the nine census regions, and the seasonal patterns observed for the 5-month period (January 1977–May 1977) were compared with the corresponding seasonal patterns of the regions to which the states belong.

Eighteen hospitals representative of census regions and bed-size categories were chosen at random, and the seasonal patterns observed for nine out of twenty-two indicators were compared with the corresponding seasonal patterns of the regions in which the hospitals are located.

The results of these validity tests are summarized below:

The seasonal patterns of states generally conform to the seasonal patterns of the census region to which the states belong. There were a few instances of nonconformity. In some states, the seasonal patterns of certain indicators, notably adult length of stay and newborn occupancy, tended to depart somewhat from regional patterns.

Generally speaking, the seasonal patterns of individual hospitals conform to the seasonal patterns of the census regions in which the hospitals are located. There were a few instances of nonconformity, and they occurred primarily for very small hospitals (under 50 beds) and very large hospitals (over 500 beds).

No validity tests were performed for metropolitan areas because data disaggregated by these areas are unavailable on a monthly basis.

Recommendations

In chapter 4 we indicated several ways in which the seasonal indexes can be used at national, regional, state, metropolitan area, and individual hospital levels. We recommend use of the regional indexes presented in tables 7-2 through 7-10 for all levels except the national level. However, because of the limited nature of the validity tests and instances of nonconformity noted, we suggest that the applicability of the regional indexes to states, metropolitan areas, or individual institutions be tested before they are put to any of the uses discussed in chapter 4. We recommend one of the following methods for testing the applicability of regional indexes.

Method 1

Using the raw data (January through December) of the desired hospital indicator pertaining to the users' specific state/metropolitan area/hospital, construct simple monthly indexes. Chapter 3 describes how these indexes may be constructed.

Plot on the same graph the simple monthly indexes and the corresponding indexes pertaining to the users' region provided in tables 7-2 through 7-10.

Examine the similiarities between the two graphs or profiles. If they are essentially similar, that is, if both graphs trace similar seesaw patterns, the regional indexes provided in this book may be used for the users' specific area of interest.[1]

Method 2

Plot the seasonal indexes of the desired hospital indicator (January through December) pertaining to the users' region from tables 7-2 through 7-10.

Plot on the same graph raw monthly data of that indicator (January through December) pertaining to the users' specific area/institution.

The user should then proceed to examine the similarities between the two graphs or profiles. Two graphs are said to be congruent to each other if they merge into one. This requires (1) that the patterns or shapes of the two graphs are identical, and (2) that the elevations of the two graphs are also identical. In the present case, one of the graphs is based on seasonal indexes and the other on raw values such as total expenses, admissions, and so on. Therefore, the elevations of the two graphs are bound to be different. In looking for similarity, the user should ignore differences in elevations, that is, heights of the graphs from the baseline, and focus on patterns or shapes. If the patterns or shapes are similar, the monthly indexes provided in this study are applicable to the users' specific area/institution.

If the foregoing tests reveal dissimilarity, the users should develop seasonal indexes of their own. See appendix II for methodology.

Note

1. Since the simple indexes make no adjustment for the trend factor, it is likely that these index values pertaining to the later part of the year would move at a slightly more elevated level than the corresponding indexes provided in this book if the hospital indicator in question has a strong upward trend. This aberration may be ignored in the case of the following hospital indications which do have a strong upward trend: total revenue, total expenses, revenue per adjusted patient day, revenue per adjusted admission, adjusted expenses per inpatient day, and adjusted expenses per admission.

Appendix I
The Nature of Time Series

A historical or longitudinal set of data is called a *time series* because it traces the movement of some measure over time. The gross national product (GNP), population, labor force, per capita income, consumer price index (CPI), and Dow Jones industrial averages are a few examples of time series we frequently hear about. So are the "Hospital Indicators," the subject matter of this study.

It may be useful to draw a distinction between absolute or volumetric time series, such as the GNP, population, total hospital expenses, patient days, and so forth, and ratio series, such as unemployment rate, per capita income, mortality rate, hospital expenses per day, occupancy rate, and so forth. Absolute time series reflect long-run growth factors such as demographic trend and economic development. Ratio series, on the other hand, reflect efficiency, productivity, capacity utilization, socioeconomic well-being, and so on.

Components

A typical time series is a composite of four elements. They are T, trend; C, cycle; S, seasonal; and I, irregular. These elements or components can be best explained with the aid of a hypothetical graph (figure AI-1).

A time series has an underlying long-term trend (T). Although we frequently

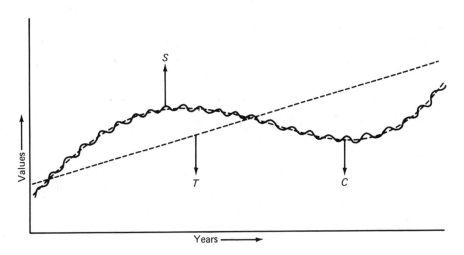

Figure AI-1. Components of a Typical Time Series

encounter time series with upward trends, there are those with downward trends as well. Energy reserves, infant mortality, and length of stay are a few examples of series with downward trends. The long-term trend of a series may be determined by fitting a trend line to historical data, as shown in figure AI-1. This may be done visually (the free-hand method) or mathematically (the least-squares method).

Cyclical oscillations (*C*) reflect business cycles which cause upswings and downswings in the volume and tempo of economic activity. The factors that give rise to business cycles are varied and complex, and have been the subject of extensive study by economists.[1] Some characteristics of business cycles deserve mention:

In business cycle terminology, the zenith of an upswing is called the *peak*, and the bottom of a downswing is called the *trough*.

They encompass a fairly long time period—sometimes as long as several years.

They do not recur with any degree of regularity. Here, for example, are the approximate dates of peaks and troughs of business cycles from 1948 to 1961.[2]

Type of swing	*Business cycle date*
Peak	November 1948
Trough	October 1949
Peak	July 1953
Trough	August 1954
Peak	July 1957
Trough	April 1958
Peak	May 1960
Trough	February 1961

The amplitude of fluctuations differs from cycle to cycle. The Great Depression of the 1930s was much more severe than anything we have encountered since then.

Certain kinds of time series are more susceptible to cyclical fluctuations than others. The GNP, industrial production, and unemployment rate, for example, are more susceptible than, say, population, patient days, and admissions.

In the health care sector, a major governmental intervention such as the introduction of Medicare and Medicaid (1966) and the Economic Stabilization Program (1971–1974) may cause oscillations approaching the amplitude and duration of business cycles.

By seasonal (S) we mean variation which recurs or repeats itself with some degree of regularity. Depending on the nature of the series, this variation could be hourly, daily, weekly, monthly, or quarterly. Climatic conditions, including variations in rainfall, cold, snow, heat, sunshine, and humidity, cause variations in demand. So do social, cultural, and institutional factors such as holidays and vacation seasons. When seasonal variations are present, the time series pertaining to an appropriate timespan, say, a year (if the variations are monthly), exhibit a seesaw pattern. For example, if we take a small segment of figure AI-1 and blow it up, we would get a graph that looks something like figure 3-1.

Most time series display a constant or stationary seasonal pattern. That is to say, the seasonal variation repeats itself with a high degree of regularity. For example, if January 1960 was a month of relatively brisk activity, this feature persists in January 1961, January 1962, and so on. The degree of constancy or regularity can be ascertained by analyzing historical data pertaining to several years. Incidentally, the hospital indicators analyzed in this study do exhibit a high degree of regularity (see chapter 5).

The fourth and final component is irregular variation (I). This is caused by a multiplicity of unpredictable factors that operate in a random fashion. Fortunately, irregular variations are relatively inconsequential. They cause, as it were, "minor wrinkles" on the graph. In addition, positive and negative variations caused by the irregular component tend to cancel each other out. Incidentally, the irregular component is ignored in figure A-1.

Notes

1. See, for example, G. Haberler, *Prosperity and Depression,* The League of Nations, Geneva, 1941; and A.F. Burns and W.C. Mitchell, *Measuring Business Cycles,* Bureau of Economic Research, New York, 1946.

2. G. Bry and C. Boschan, *Cyclical Analysis of Time Series: Selected Procedures and Computer Programs,* National Bureau of Economic Research, New York, 1971, p. 54. Reproduced with permission.

Appendix II
Development of Seasonal
Indexes

It is possible to separate out the constituent elements of a given time series. The process is called *time-series decomposition* and is discussed in detail in most textbooks on statistics.[1] In this appendix we will describe briefly how the monthly indexes of hospital indicators were developed.

We have seen in Appendix I that if we ignore irregular variation (I), a time series may be thought of as a composite of *TCS,* or $T \times C \times S$. A 12-month moving average is considered an estimate of $T \times C$ because the moving average smoothes out seasonal variations. Consequently, if we divide the original data by the 12-month moving averages, we have an estimate of seasonal movements, that is,

$$\frac{T \times C \times S}{T \times C} = S$$

Using historical data on admissions as an example, a step-by-step description of the procedure employed in this study is set forth below:

1. Monthly data on admissions for the 14-year period—January 1963 through December 1976—are displayed in figure AII-1. Notice that the thin jagged line representing raw data vividly depicts the monthly fluctuations present in the series.

2. We now proceed to calculate the centered 12-month moving average. The steps involved are as follows:

(a) Compute the 13-month moving weighted total for July 1963, August 1963, and so on as follows:

July 1963 = 1(Jan. 63) + 2(Feb. 63) + $\cdots$ + 2(Dec. 64) + 1(Jan. 64)

Aug. 1963 = 1(Feb. 63) + 2(Mar. 63) + $\cdots$ + 2(Jan. 64) + 1(Feb. 64)

(b) Obtain the centered 12-month moving average by dividing the values obtained in (a) above by 24.

The double line in figure AII-1 represents the centered 12-month moving average. Notice that the moving average smoothes out seasonal and irregular components but retains the trend and cycle components.

121

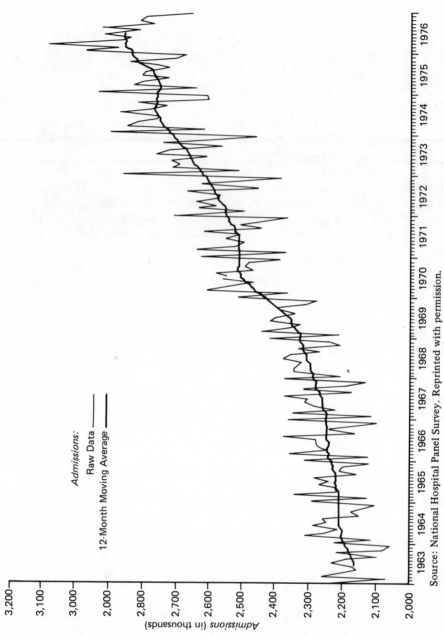

Source: National Hospital Panel Survey. Reprinted with permission.

Figure AII-1. Admissions: Raw Data and 12-Month Moving Average, January 1963–December 1976

3. The seasonal factor for each month is obtained by dividing the raw monthly value by the corresponding centered 12-month moving average. Table AII-1 displays the computational layout for a segment of the data. For example, the original value for January 1970 is 2,523,00 admissions. The centered 12-month moving average for the same period is 2,433,000 admissions. Thus the seasonal factor for January 1970 is[2]

$$\frac{2,523,000}{2,433,000} = 1.033$$

4. Having computed the seasonal factors for all months in the data set, a table of monthly arrays is set up. Each column of this table will have the seasonal factors pertaining to all Januarys, all Februarys, and so on. Table AII-2 shows the results of this procedure for admissions. Note that the figures obtained in the last column of table AII-1 appear on table AII-2 in the line for 1970. No values appear for January through June 1963 and July through December 1976, for 6 months' data both prior to and past a given month must be available to compute the moving average. This is also apparent in figure AII-1.

Table AII-1
Admissions, 1970

Period, 1970	1 Admissions (thousands)	2 13-Month Moving Total Weighted 1,2,2,...,2,2,1	3 Centered 12-Month Moving Average (Col. 2 ÷ 24)	4 Percent of 12-Month Moving Average (Col. 1 ÷ Col. 3)
January	2,523	58,627	2,443	1.033
February	2,367	59,029	2,460	0.962
March	2,618	59,365	2,474	1.058
April	2,537	59,554	2,481	1.022
May	2,480	59,832	2,493	0.994
June	2,572	60,131	2,505	1.026
July	2,560	60,364	2,515	1.017
August	2,596	60,487	2,520	1.030
September	2,479	60,542	2,523	0.982
October	2,505	60,581	2,524	0.992
November	2,491	60,606	2,525	0.986
December	2,398	60,629	2,526	0.949

Source: National Hospital Panel Survey. Reprinted with permission.

Table AII-2
Seasonal Adjustment Factors, Admissions

Year	Jan.	Feb.	Mar.	Apr.	May	June	July	Aug.	Sept.	Oct.	Nov.	Dec.	Mean
1963	0.0000	0.0000	0.0000	0.0000	0.0000	0.0000	1.0316	1.0113	0.9623	1.0208	0.9495	0.9362	
1964	1.0417	0.9641	1.0501	1.0205	1.0022	1.0364	1.0152	1.0228	0.9672	0.9836	0.9690	0.9485	
1965	1.0378	0.9609	1.0585	0.9995	0.9991	1.0216	1.0063	1.0296	0.9682	0.9929	0.9859	0.9484	
1966	1.0352	0.9463	1.0512	0.9974	1.0122	1.0162	1.0154	1.0577	0.9625	0.9970	0.9663	0.9332	
1967	1.0541	0.9425	1.0447	0.9859	1.0084	1.0237	1.0180	1.0492	0.9575	1.0187	0.9616	0.9272	
1968	1.0410	0.9603	1.0476	1.0210	1.0153	1.0069	1.0314	1.0208	0.9774	1.0026	0.9492	0.9636	
1969	1.0394	0.9445	1.0476	1.0092	0.9882	1.0280	1.0174	0.9864	1.0011	0.9989	0.9572	0.9360	
1970	1.0330	0.9625	1.0585	1.0225	0.9947	1.0263	1.0177	1.0300	0.9827	0.9925	0.9863	0.9491	
1971	1.0434	0.9426	1.0542	1.0036	0.9934	1.0175	0.9956	1.0403	0.9666	0.9941	0.9701	0.9270	
1972	1.0641	0.9761	1.0293	1.0084	1.0331	1.0027	0.9953	1.0310	0.9450	1.0137	0.9701	0.9143	
1973	1.0926	0.9539	1.0296	1.0161	1.0236	0.9800	1.0357	1.0206	0.9521	1.0209	0.9704	0.9069	
1974	1.0675	0.9568	1.0418	1.0258	1.0090	1.0026	1.0389	1.0069	0.9877	1.0183	0.9434	0.9446	
1975	1.0652	0.9585	1.0293	1.0177	0.9839	1.0139	1.0087	0.9781	0.9839	1.0125	0.9566	0.9411	
1976	1.0476	1.0096	1.0795	1.0050	0.9948	1.0196	0.0000	0.0000	0.0000	0.0000	0.0000	0.0000	
Total Excluding Outliers	11.5370	10.5265	11.4948	11.1209	11.0409	11.1790	11.1930	11.2489	10.6681	11.0620	10.6059	10.3056	
Modified Mean	1.0488	0.9570	1.0450	1.0110	1.0037	1.0163	1.0175	1.0226	0.9698	1.0056	0.9642	0.9369	0.9999
Seasonal Index Modified Mean × (1/0.9999)	1.0490	0.9571	1.0451	1.0111	1.0039	1.0164	1.0177	1.0228	0.9700	1.0058	0.9643	0.9370	1.0000
Standard Deviation	0.0170	0.0173	0.0154	0.0109	0.0137	0.0137	0.0137	0.0216	0.0148	0.0126	0.0130	0.0148	
95 Percent Conf. Int. (S.D. × 1.96)	0.0332	0.0337	0.0302	0.0215	0.0269	0.0269	0.0269	0.0423	0.0289	0.0246	0.0254	0.0289	

5. The constancy or stability of the seasonal factors is then examined. If the individual arrays are widely dispersed (that is, cover a wide range of values vertically), we can have little confidence in the seasonal indexes. The less the dispersion of individual monthly arrays, the more stable or constant is the seasonal movement from year to year. An estimate of stability is obtained by computing the standard deviation of each monthly array. The smaller the standard deviation, the greater the stability, and vice versa. The standard deviation for each month is presented on the bottom line of table AII-2.

6. From each monthly array, two extreme values (the highest and the lowest) are dropped. These figures are circled in table AII-2. An average of the remaining values, the *modified mean,* is then computed. This average is the unadjusted seasonal index for that month.

7. The averages obtained in the preceding step for the months of January through December are subjected to a minor adjustment to ensure that the sum of the averages, when divided by 12, works out to 1.000. This is done by adjusting each month's modified mean by a factor. Turning to the last column of table AII-2, the average of the modified means is 0.9999, which falls short of 1.0000 by 0.0001. In order to correct this discrepancy, each month's modified mean is multiplied by $1 \div 0.9999 = 1.0001$. These adjusted averages, labeled *seasonal index* in table AII-2, are the indexes presented in this study.

Notes

1. See, for example, F.E. Croxton and D.J. Cowden, *Applied General Statistics,* Prentice-Hall, New Jersey, 1963, chaps. 11, 12, 13, 14, 15, and 16.

2. The original calculations were, of course, performed with unrounded numbers.

Glossary

A glossary of indicators traditionally used in the hospital system, including their interrelations, appears below. In most cases, more than one formula is presented. In these cases, the first formula is more meaningful in the sense that it brings out the significance of the indicator more clearly. However, the alternative formulas are useful for three reasons. First, they provide a means of looking at the indicator from a different perspective. Second, they help one's understanding of how changes in certain indicators affect other indicators. Finally, they may also have some computational advantages. For example, in situations where data on a certain element of the formula are unavailable, alternative formulas may be used to derive the desired indicators. In general, formulas involving length of stay (LOS) and occupancy rate (OR) tend to be less accurate because of rounding errors.

It is assumed that the indicators are computed from the data pertaining to 1 year. If the data pertain to periods other than a year, the value 365, wherever it appears, should be replaced by appropriate values.

Abbreviations

A = admissions

A_{65} = admissions: 65 and over

AA = adjusted admissions

$AADC$ = adjusted average daily census

ADC_n = average daily census: newborn

AEA = adjusted expenses per admission

AED = adjusted expenses per inpatient day

AEV = adjusted expenses per outpatient visit

APD = adjusted patient days

$ATOR$ = adjusted patient turnover rate

B = beds

BAS = bassinets

BIR = births

D = discharges

D_{65} = discharges: 65 and over

D_n = discharges: newborn

EC = excess capacity

IPR = inpatient revenue

LOS = length of stay: adult

LOS_{65} = length of stay: 65 and over

LOS_n = length of stay: newborn

OPR = outpatient revenue

OPV = outpatient visits

OR = occupancy rate

OR_n = occupancy rate: newborn

PD = patient days

PD_{65} = patient days: 65 and over

PD_n = patient days: newborn

$ROPV$ = revenue per outpatient visit

RPA = revenue per admission

RPD = revenue per inpatient day

TE = total expenses

TOR = turnover rate: inpatient

TPR = total patient revenue

Formulas

$$A = PD/LOS = (ADC \times 365)/LOS = D^*$$

$$A_{65} = PD_{65}/LOS_{65} = D^*_{65}$$

$$AA = A + OPV\left(\frac{ROPV}{RPA}\right) = A + A\left(\frac{OPR}{IPR}\right) = A\left(\frac{TPR}{IPR}\right)$$

$$AADC = APD/365$$

$$ADC = PD/365 = (A \times LOS)/365$$

$$AEA = \frac{TE}{AA} = \frac{TE\left(\frac{IPR}{TPR}\right)}{A} = \frac{TE \times IPR}{A(TPR)} = \frac{TE}{A + A\left(\frac{OPR}{IPR}\right)}$$

$$= \frac{TE}{A\left(\frac{TPR}{IPR}\right)}$$

$$AED = \frac{TE}{APD} = \frac{TE\left(\frac{IPR}{TPR}\right)}{PD} = \frac{TE \times IPR}{PD(TPR)}$$

$$= \frac{TE}{PD + PD\left(\frac{OPR}{IPR}\right)} = \frac{TE}{PD\left(\frac{TPR}{IPR}\right)}$$

$$AEV = \frac{TE\left(\frac{OPR}{TPR}\right)}{OPV} = \frac{TE}{OPV + PD\left(\frac{RPD}{ROPV}\right)} = \frac{TE \times OPR}{OPV(TPR)}$$

$$= \frac{TE}{OPV\left(\frac{TPR}{OPR}\right)}$$

$$APD = PD + OPV\left(\frac{ROPV}{RPD}\right) = PD\left(\frac{TPR}{IPR}\right) = PD\left(1 + \frac{OPR}{IPR}\right)$$

$$ATOR\dagger = \frac{AA}{B} = \frac{A\left(1 + \frac{OPR}{TPR}\right)}{B}$$

$$D = A^* = PD/LOS$$

$$D_{65} = A_{65}^* = PD_{65}/LOS_{65}$$

$$D_n = A_n^* = PD_n/LOS_n$$

$$EC = 1 - OR = 1 - [PD/(B \times 365)]$$

$$LOS = PD/D = PD/A$$

$$LOS_{65} = PD_{65}/D_{65} = PD_{65}/A_{65}$$

$$LOS_n = PD_n/BIR$$

$$OR = ADC/B = PD/(B \times 365)$$

$$OR_n = ADC_n/BAS = PD_n/(BAS \times 365)$$

$$PD = (ADC \times 365) = (A \times LOS) = (B \times OR \times 365)$$

$$PD_{65} = (A_{65} \times LOS_{65})$$

$$PD_n = BIR \times LOS_n$$

$$TOR = \frac{A}{B} = \frac{PD/LOS}{PD/(OR \times 365)} = \frac{(OR \times 365)}{LOS}$$

---

*Admissions (A) approximate discharges (D) in short-term hospitals.

†Adjusted turnover rate ($ATOR$) is called "hospital utilization index" in Hospital Administrative Services Program (see *HAS Six-Month National Data for Period Ending June 30, 1977,* AHA, Chicago, 1977, p. 7.

References

American Hospital Association, *Hospital Statistics* (various issues), Chicago.

American Hospital Association, *Hospitals,* Journal of the American Hospital Association (various issues).

American Hospital Association, *Comparative Statistics of Health Facilities and Population: Metropolitan and Nonmetropolitan Areas,* Chicago, 1978, p. 20.

V.P. Barabba, "Population Trends and the Cost of Medical Care," *U.S. Dept. of Commerce News,* Washington, July 20, 1976.

M.S. Beauliew, "Dual Purpose OB Unit: Alice Peck Day Memorial Hospital, Lebanon, New Hampshire," *Hospital Topics* (May 1966): 118-119.

G. Bry and C. Boschan, *Cyclical Analysis of Time Series: Selected Procedures and Computer Programs,* National Bureau of Economic Research, New York, 1971, p. 54.

A.F. Burns and W.C. Mitchell, *Measuring Business Cycles,* Bureau of Economic Analysis, New York, 1946.

K. Change, S. Chan, W. Low, and C. Ng, "Climate and Conception Rates in Hong Kong," *Human Biol.* 35 (Sept. 1963).

"College, ASA Release Surgical Study Findings," *Bulletin of the Amer. Coll. of Surgeons* 60 (July 1975):4.

Commission on Prof. and Hosp. Activities, *Length of Stay in PAS Hospitals, by Diagnosis, United States, 1975,* Ann Arbor, Oct. 1971.

Council on Wage and Price Stability, *The Complex Puzzle of Rising Health Care Costs: Can the Private Sector Fit It Together?* Washington, Dec. 1976, p. 73.

F.E. Croxton and D.J. Cowden, *Applied General Statistics,* Prentice-Hall, New Jersey, 1963, chaps. 11, 12, 13, 14, 15, and 16.

S. Falk, "Average Length of Stay in Long-Term Institutions," *Health Services Research* 6 (Fall 1971):251-55.

"Feasibility of a 5-Day Medical-Surgical Unit," *Hospital Administration Currents* 21 (Jan.-Feb. 1977):1-4.

M. Feldstein and A. Taylor, *The Rapid Rise of Hospital Costs,* Council on Wage and Price Stability, Staff Report, Washington, January 1977, pp. 24-28.

F. Gordon, "Why Not Join Surgery with the Obstetric Unit," *Modern Hospital* (Aug. 1967):115-118.

M. Gornick, "Medicare Patients: Geographic Differences in Hospital Discharge Rates and Multiple Stays," *Social Security Bulletin* (June 1977):28.

Haberler, G. *Prosperity and Depression,* The League of Nations, Geneva, 1941.

National Academy of Science, *Controlling the Supply of Hospital Beds; A Policy Statement,* Institute of Medicine, Washington, 1976.

"National Guidelines for Health Planning," *Federal Register* 43 (Mar. 1978):13040-50.

B. Pasamanick, S. Danitz, and H. Knoblock, "Socio-Economic and Seasonal Variations in Birth Rates," *Milbank Memo. Fund Quart.* 38 (July 1960).

P.J. Phillip, "HCI/HII—Two New AHA Indexes Measure Costs, Intensity," *Hospital Fin. Management* (April 1977):20-26.

P.J. Phillip, "New AHA Indexes Provide Fairer View of Rising Costs". *Hospitals* (July 16, 1977):175-182.

P.J. Phillip, "Some Considerations Involved in Determining the Optimum Size of Specialized Hospital Facilities," *Inquiry* IV (Dec. 1969):44-48.

P.J. Phillip, R. Foster, J. Jeffers, and A. Hai, *The Nature of Hospital Costs: Three Studies,* Hospital Research and Educational Trust, Chicago, 1976, pp. 200-262.

E. Takahashi, "Seasonal Variations of Conception and Suicide," *Tohoku J. of Experimental Medicine* 84 (December 1964).

U.S. Bureau of Census, *Current Population Reports,* Series P-23, No. 43, U.S. Govt. Printing Office, Washington, 1973.

U.S. Department of Health, Education and Welfare, *Health, United States, 1976-77,* DHEW Pub. No. (HRA)77-1232, Public Health Service, Washington, p. 215.

U.S. Department of Health, Education and Welfare, *Selected Charge Patterns in Short-Stay Hospitals under Medicare,* No. HI-31, SSA, Washington, Sept. 30, 1971, Chart B.

U.S. Dept. of Labor, *Chartbook on Prices, Wages, and Productivity,* Bureau of Labor Statistics, Washington, May 1977, p. 1.

Index

About the Authors

Stephen Dombrosk is the coauthor of a study of hospital closures published in *Hospitals* magazine, and of *Selected Community Hospital Indicators, 1977.* He was a participant in the Third Illinois Health Care Research Symposium. At George Washington University he studied public affairs and received the B.A. in economics from the University of Connecticut. Currently he works as a research assistant at the American Hospital Association.

P.J. Phillip, a native of India, received the B.A. and M.A. degrees in economics from the University of Poona (India), the M.B.A. from the University of Detroit, and the Ph.D. in educational statistics from Wayne State University. Dr. Phillip has served as research planning consultant for Michigan Blue Cross, and research director for the Blue Cross Association. Currently he is the director, Hospital Research Center, Office of Research Affairs, American Hospital Association.

Dr. Phillip has published several papers in professional journals, and presented papers in national and international symposia. He is the coauthor of *Factors Affecting Staffing Levels and Patterns of Nursing Personnel* (Government Printing Office, Washington, D.C., 1975); *A Taxonomy of Community Hospitals* (American Hospital Association, Chicago, 1975); and *The Nature of Hospital Costs: Three Studies* (Hospital Research and Educational Trust, Chicago, 1976).